NUTRITION AND HEALTH

FOOD ALLERGIES

A GROWING PROBLEM

BY JASON BRAINARD

Portions of this book originally appeared in *Food Allergies* by Kevin Hillstrom.

LUCENT PRESS

Published in 2020 by
Lucent Press, an Imprint of Greenhaven Publishing, LLC
353 3rd Avenue
Suite 255
New York, NY 10010

Designer: Deanna Paternostro
Editor: Jennifer Lombardo

Library of Congress Cataloging-in-Publication Data

Names: Brainard, Jason, author.
Title: Food allergies : a growing problem / Jason Brainard.
Description: New York : Lucent Press, c2020. | Series: Diseases and disorders | Includes bibliographical references and index.
Identifiers: LCCN 2019019592 (print) | LCCN 2019022398 (ebook) | ISBN 9781534568709 (library bound book) | ISBN 9781534568761 (pbk. book)
Subjects: LCSH: Food allergy–Popular works.
Classification: LCC RC596 .B7245 2020 (print) | LCC RC596 (ebook) | DDC 616.97/5–dc23
LC record available at https://lccn.loc.gov/2019019592
LC ebook record available at https://lccn.loc.gov/2019022398

Printed in China

CPSIA compliance information: Batch #BW20KL: For further information contact Greenhaven Publishing LLC, New York, New York at 1-844-317-7404.

Please visit our website, www.greenhavenpublishing.com. For a free color catalog of all our high-quality books, call toll free 1-844-317-7404 or fax 1-844-317-7405.

CONTENTS

FOREWORD

People often want to do whatever they can to live healthy lives, but this is frequently easier said than done. For example, experts suggest minimizing stress as it takes a long-term toll on the body and mind. However, in an era where young adults must balance school attendance, extracurricular and social activities, and several hours of homework each night, stress is virtually unavoidable. Socioeconomic factors also come into play, which can prevent someone from making good health choices even when they are aware of what the consequences will be.

Other times, however, the problem is misinformation. The media frequently reports watered-down versions of scientific findings, distorting the message and causing confusion. Sometimes multiple conflicting results are reported, leaving people to wonder whether a simple action such as eating dark chocolate is helpful, harmful, or has no effect on their health at all. In such an environment, many people ignore all health news and decide for themselves what the best course of action is. This has led to dangerous trends such as the recent anti-vaccination movement.

The titles in the Nutrition and Health series aim to give young adults the information they need to take charge of their health. Factual, unbiased text presents all sides of current health issues with the understanding that everyone is different and knows their own body and health needs best. Readers also gain insight into important nutrition topics, such as whether a vegetarian diet is right for them, which foods may improve or exacerbate any existing health issues, and precautions they can take to prevent the spread of foodborne illnesses.

Annotated quotes from medical experts provide accurate and accessible explanations of challenging concepts, as well as different points of view on controversial issues. Additional books and websites are listed, giving readers a starting point from which to delve deeper into specific topics that are of interest to them. Full-color photographs, fact boxes, and enlightening charts are presented alongside the informative text to give young adults a clearer picture of today's most pressing health concerns.

With so much complicated and conflicting information about nutrition and health available on social media and in the news, it can be hard for all people—but especially for young adults—to make smart choices about their health. However, this series presents an accessible approach to health education that makes the work of staying healthy seem much less intimidating.

Introduction

FOOD SAFETY AND ALLERGIES

Everyone needs to eat, and in fact, eating can be one of life's greatest pleasures. However, for many people, eating can be hard work that is worrisome and even dangerous. While some people do not like broccoli, others choose not to eat meat, and others may need to limit salt in their diet, a growing group of people have to worry about becoming violently ill if they eat the wrong thing. For those with food allergies, a meal prepared with the wrong ingredients could end with them covered in swollen hives, having diarrhea or vomiting—or in the worst cases, dying.

People with food allergies account for a relatively small percentage of the U.S. population. Scientists and doctors generally agree that about 32 million Americans live with food allergies. This figure includes about 8 percent of all American kids. The number of Americans with food allergies is rising quickly, and researchers worry that it is emerging as a major public health issue. Furthermore, the most common food allergens are not rare and exotic. They are found everywhere. Those with food allergies must remain vigilant.

The impact of food allergies is already being felt in many areas of American society. Millions of families are restructuring their daily lives to keep family members with food allergies safe from harm. Schools, summer camps, and day-care centers are rewriting their snack and lunch rules to keep peanuts, milk, eggs, and other allergenic foods far away from their students and campers. Children and teens are educating themselves about what they should do if a friend with food allergies has a serious allergic reaction.

The biggest life adjustments, though, have to be undertaken by the people who actually live with food allergies every day. This task can be

A Closer Look

Some allergic reactions resolve themselves on their own. Others are severe enough to require medical attention.

enormously challenging, especially if they have life-threatening reactions to certain foods. People with severe food allergies have to take precautions to avoid even trace, or tiny, amounts of peanuts, milk, wheat, shellfish, and other common food items that are deadly to them.

People with allergies constantly have to think about the ingredients in the foods they eat. For example, many types of cake and frosting are made with milk, so someone who is allergic to dairy may not be able to eat them, depending on how severe their allergy is.

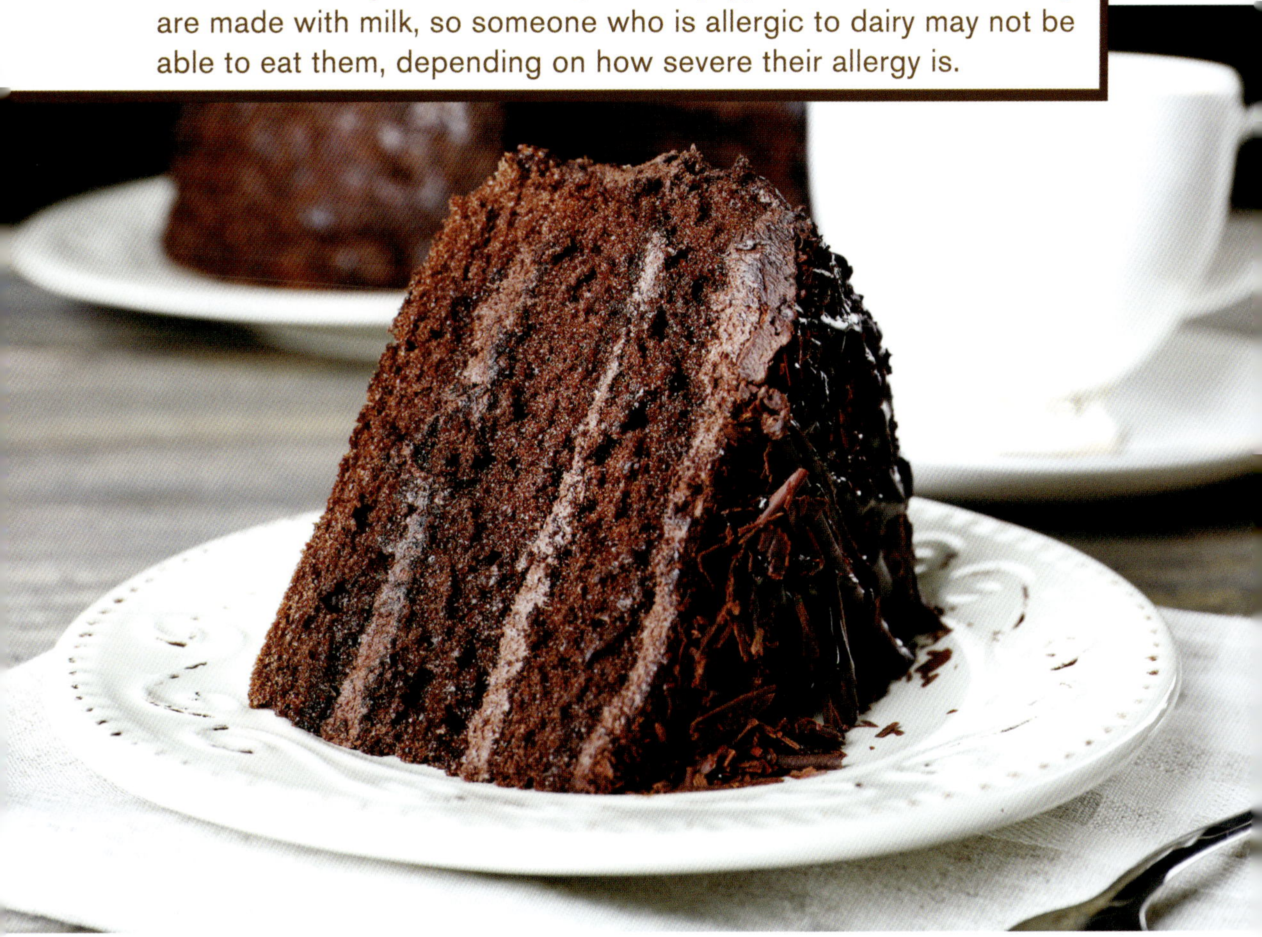

Nonetheless, millions of men, women, and children who have serious food allergies have managed to find other foods that are both nutritious and tasty. They also lead fun and fulfilling lives. Sandra Beasley is an award-winning poet who has allergies to dairy (including goat's milk), egg, soy, beef, shrimp, pine nuts, cucumbers, cantaloupe, honeydew, mango, macadamia nuts, pistachios, swordfish, and mustard. She is also allergic to mold, dust, grass and tree pollen, dogs, rabbits, cigarette smoke, horses, and wool. Beasley agrees that all of these allergies have made life more complicated for her and her friends and family, but she also has a successful writing career and a vibrant circle of friends. "Those with food allergies aren't victims," she said. "We're people who—for better or for worse—experience the world in a slightly different way."[1]

Chapter One

DEFINING FOOD ALLERGIES

More than 50 million children in the United States head off to school every weekday. Most of these students look forward to their lunch each day. Lunch can be a welcome break from the expectations of teachers and a time to visit with friends. Some students open up meals brought from home, while others buy their lunch from the cafeteria. Most do not give a second thought to the safety of their meal.

For kids such as Caleigh, though, lunchtime is a potentially dangerous part of the day. Caleigh was diagnosed with a serious peanut and tree nut allergy when she was a baby. As a result, Caleigh's elementary school adopted a wide range of policies to protect her from accidental exposure to nuts. Some of Caleigh's friends and classmates probably do not fully understand why all these special rules are in place. A number of their parents may even feel annoyed or frustrated about these measures. They may think it is unnecessary for them to take precautions when their own children are not the ones who have allergies.

These rules may seem silly to most people, but they are put in place for a good reason: to protect children such as Caleigh. For example, if someone with a peanut butter sandwich gets some peanut butter on the table and Caleigh later sits at that table and gets peanut butter on her own food, she will become ill and could potentially die if help is not given to her in time. It is difficult for people without allergies to understand how something as simple as a sandwich could be so dangerous.

The Immune System and Allergic Reactions

Most allergic reactions are not life-threatening. In most people, exposure

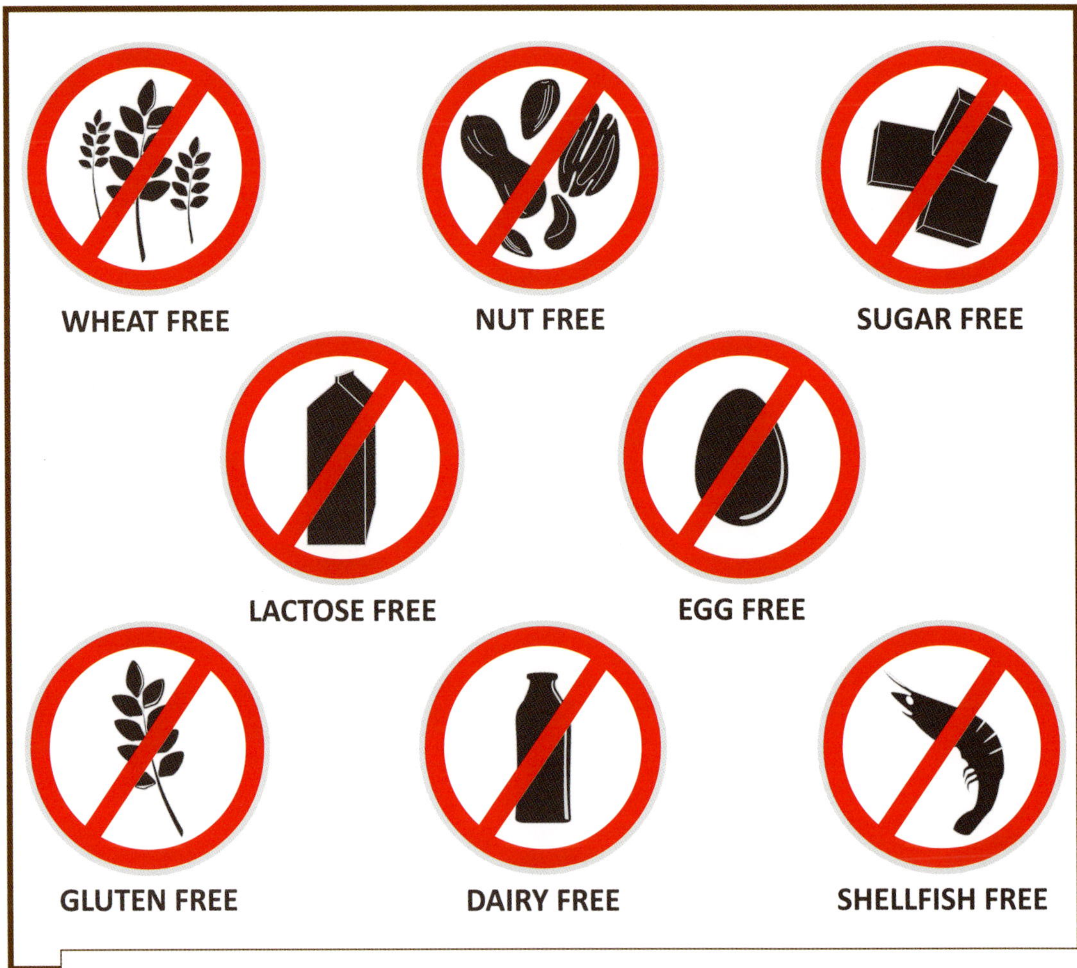

People with allergies need to carefully read the packaging of the foods they buy. If a package does not clearly say it has no allergens in it, someone with a food allergy should be cautious.

to a food allergen will cause a variety of symptoms that are unpleasant but non-deadly, including a rash, hives, itchy skin, sneezing, stomach cramps, and increased difficulty breathing or speaking. For some, though, exposure to an allergen can cause symptoms that will kill them if they are not treated immediately. The severity of an allergy varies from person to person, and there is no way to tell by looking at someone how severe their allergy is.

The immune system is a wonderfully complex and hardworking part of the human body. It serves as the first line of defense against germs and diseases. The immune system creates antibodies, which are proteins that destroy bacteria, viruses, and other microorganisms that can make people sick when they enter the body. Food allergies occur, though, when a person's immune system misidentifies healthy food proteins as a threat—such as a harmful virus—and mobilizes antibodies to wipe out that threat. In the worst of these cases of mistaken identity, the immune system works so furiously to destroy the innocent food proteins that it does severe or fatal damage to the body it is trying to protect. This same misidentification accounts for allergic reactions to harmless things such as penicillin, pollen, and dogs. In other words, as the website KidsHealth explained, "the thing itself isn't harmful, but the way your body reacts to it is."[2]

Scientists and scholars have described this phenomenon in a variety of ways. Robert A. Wood is a children's allergist at Johns Hopkins University School of Medicine. He compared food allergies to overprotective parents by saying, "Trying too hard to do the best for their children, they often cause more harm."[3] Science writer Laura Beil compared a person's immune system to the staff at a busy restaurant. When peanuts or other common allergenic substances—known as allergens—enter the digestive system after being eaten, they are first greeted by cells that work like a restaurant hostess. These cells escort guests (the allergens) to their table and alert the waiters. Beil continued,

> *The waiters … are the T cells, which help the body recognize friend from foe. When food allergy develops, the T cells, instead of welcoming the peanut as the valued customer it is, initiate a process that alerts another type of immune cell, called a B cell. B cells make antibodies—the body's bouncers. In the case of food allergies, B cells start to make IgE [immunoglobulin E] antibodies, which when bound to a peanut protein summon mast cells. Mast cells come armed with chemical weapons. Substances released from mast cells, including histamines and cytokines, lead to the most frightening symptoms of food allergies: hives, vomiting, and anaphylaxis [a severe allergic reaction that afflicts the entire body], which can be deadly. Once the IgE antibodies are on patrol, the peanut protein finds itself on the blacklist, and will be violently ejected by security should it try to return.*[4]

A Closer Look

According to a 2018 report published by Blue Cross Blue Shield health insurance, emergency room visits to treat anaphylaxis in children increased by 150 percent between 2010 and 2016. A majority of the patients were treated for exposure to peanuts or tree nuts.

The Problem with Lying About Allergies

Some people with reactions to certain foods have such mild symptoms that they continue to eat that particular food anyway; for example, someone whose lips and tongue itch slightly when they eat strawberries may decide they like strawberries more than they dislike experiencing these symptoms. This is generally considered a sensitivity or intolerance rather than a "true" allergy, but many people are unaware of this distinction between the terms. A person with a true strawberry allergy may break out in hives all over their body and have difficulty breathing, making it both unpleasant and dangerous for them to keep eating this food.

Because two people may have very different reactions to the same food but call both of them an allergy, someone may assume one of them is lying. Further complicating the issue is the fact that some people do lie about having an allergy. Most people who do this are trying to avoid a food they dislike. For example, someone who dislikes walnuts may think saying they have an allergy is a more polite way to refuse the nut-filled brownies their friend made than simply saying they do not want to eat the brownies. Others who lie do so because they have an eating disorder and are trying to avoid eating without letting their friends know why. Although most people are not trying to hurt anyone, this type of lie can have multiple negative consequences. First, "telling people you're actually allergic to the food may seem like an easy way out, but in reality

Symptoms of a Food Allergy

When histamines are released into the body, many physical changes occur. Histamine is a chemical that triggers blood vessels to expand. This gets blood and immune cells to the site of the threat—or, in the case of allergies, the false threat—more quickly. As a result, blood floods the affected area, causing redness and swelling. This is known as inflammation or an inflammatory response, and it is why a person's lips and tongue may swell when they eat a food they are allergic to. An inflammatory response has other effects as well. It causes the smooth muscles in the airways to constrict, which leads to wheezing and difficulty

it makes others work hard to accommodate you and your special diet."[1] Second, if the person later reveals that they were lying or eats the food they say they are allergic to anyway, it creates a mistrust of anyone who says they have an allergy. This can have dangerous consequences for a person with a severe allergy because if a person who prepares their food assumes they are lying, they may not be as careful as they should be about keeping the allergen out of the person's food. In an article for *Cosmopolitan* magazine, editor Lane Moore explained:

> *Listen, I honestly, truly do not care if you just don't like eating whatever food or you try to stay away from it because you don't feel that great when you eat it … But saying you have an allergy, while everyone knows you don't have one, just puts me on trial every time I have to tell someone … I have to convince waiters, who will often lie about the ingredients in foods and tell me my allergens aren't in there when they are, and then I end up vomiting all night or with a full body rash or my throat swelling up like it's full of golf ball-size grenades. Basically, I have to prove I'm not like you.*[2]

1. Jill Castle, "Why People Claim to Have Food Allergies," Verywell Health, last updated May 19, 2018. www.verywellhealth.com/fake-food-allergies-1323997.

2. Lane Moore, "Stop Lying About Having Food Allergies," *Cosmopolitan*, December 3, 2014. www.cosmopolitan.com/sex-love/news/a33064/people-lying-about-food-allergies/.

breathing, and it prompts the body to try to expel harmful substances in the form of sneezing, coughing, vomiting, and diarrhea. It is the release of histamine and the accompanying inflammatory response that defines an allergic reaction. It is this reaction, not the allergen itself, that makes people feel ill. In addition, people who experience severe allergic reactions to food often feel a sense of approaching doom when their allergy attack begins. As journalist Susan Dominus explained, "People in early stages of a reaction often feel profoundly that something is very, very wrong, just as they feel the first hints of an itch."[5]

Allergic reactions to food generally occur within an hour or two of eating. The more severe reactions, though, often happen more quickly. Serious reactions frequently trigger symptoms within a minute or two of contact with the allergenic food. Sometimes symptoms even appear within a matter of seconds.

People with severe allergies to certain foods do not always have to eat that food to experience an allergic reaction; it can happen when they simply touch or breathe in particles of the food. For example, teenager Stone Cofini from New York is so allergic to peanuts that he could have a deadly reaction just from inhaling peanut dust. This is why many places have made rules restricting what foods can be brought into an area where a person with an allergy works, plays, or attends school.

In 2016, several news outlets reported the story of 20-year-old Myriam Ducré-Lemay, whose peanut allergy proved fatal for her in 2012. Myriam's new boyfriend, who was unaware of her allergy, ate a peanut butter sandwich, brushed his teeth, and then kissed Myriam goodnight. Even this small amount of contact was enough to give Myriam an allergic reaction, and although she was rushed to the hospital, she soon died. However, this was a very rare tragedy. A similar story was reported in 2005 concerning a girl named Christina Desforges, but in that case, it was later proven that nine hours had passed between the time Christina's boyfriend ate peanuts and the time he kissed her. This was enough time for the body to completely remove the allergen from his saliva. A medical examiner determined that Christina's true cause of death was an asthma attack.

Anaphylaxis

Minor food allergies involve only one or two symptoms. More serious reactions, though, can affect multiple organ systems, including the skin, respiratory system, digestive system, and cardiovascular system. When this happens, the reaction is called anaphylaxis. It generally begins with hives (raised welts on the skin), the swelling of the tongue and throat, and breathing problems. If anaphylaxis is not controlled, it causes a dangerous drop in blood pressure that produces shock. When an individual goes into anaphylactic shock, blood pressure drops and the brain and other vital organs are starved of oxygen. Death can result within minutes of going into shock.

Anaphylactic shock can unfold in three different ways. In a uniphasic attack, the allergic person experiences a single wave of

Hives (shown here) are one result of anaphylaxis. They appear on the skin when histamine causes blood plasma to leak out of small blood vessels in the skin.

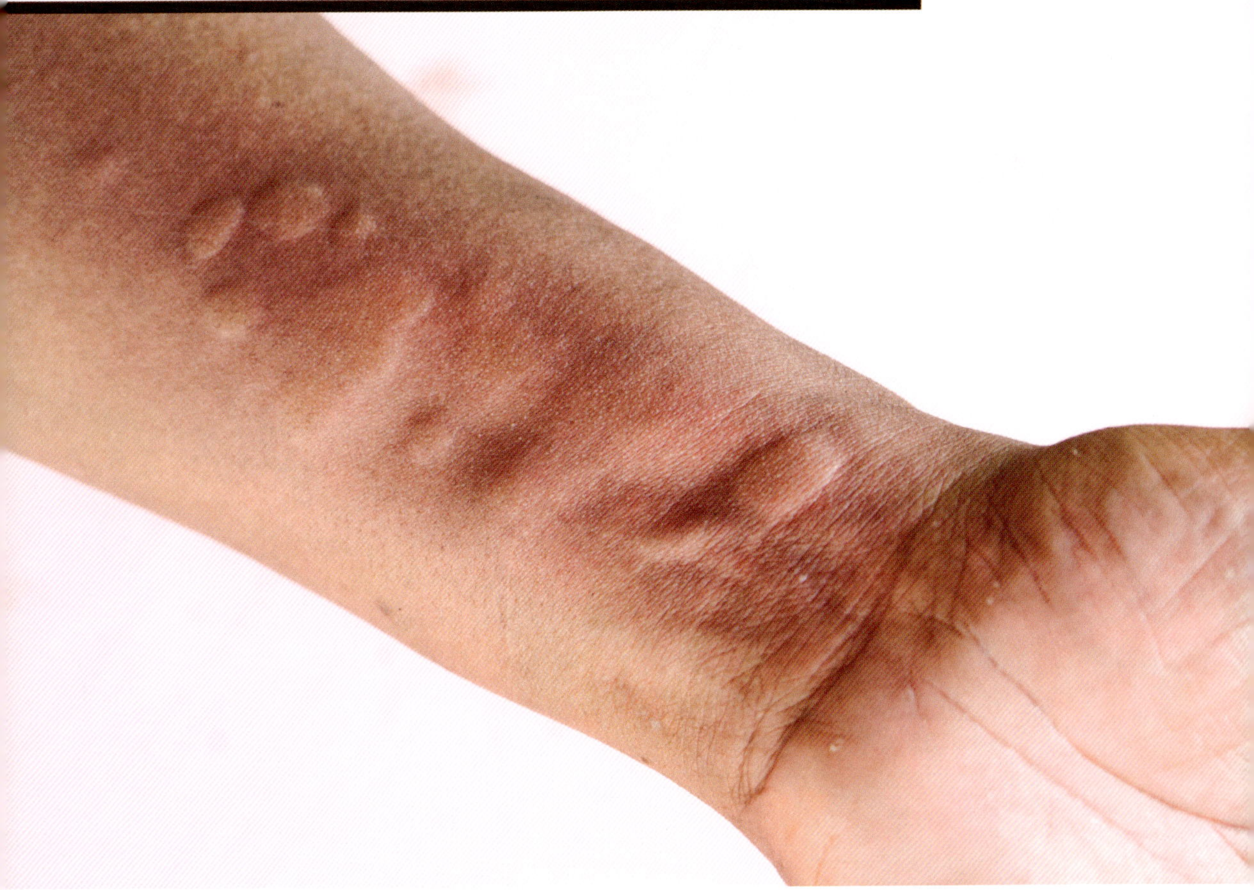

symptoms. The majority of anaphylactic shock episodes are uniphasic in nature. Another 20 percent or so of attacks are biphasic, which means that the individual suffers a second wave of symptoms after the initial reaction has faded. Finally, anaphylactic shock will occasionally take what is known as a protracted form. In these situations, severe allergic symptoms remain for up to 48 hours, even with treatment.

Anaphylactic shock is an extremely scary event for people with allergies as well as their families and friends. Some people with food allergies who have gone into anaphylactic shock say that even after they recover physically, the memory of the event can still scare them. Dean is a young man who nearly died from anaphylactic shock after eating a peanut butter cookie. He said, "I lost 25 pounds right after it happened because I just … didn't eat. I was afraid to eat. I suddenly realized there were nuts everywhere." Dean has since regained some of that weight, but he admitted, "I'm still nervous all the time. I think about it every time I sit down to eat. I feel a lack of confidence."[6]

Anaphylaxis, as opposed to isolated milder symptoms such as watery eyes and an itchy throat, generally occurs when a person with severe allergies accidentally eats something with the allergenic food in it, rather than breathing it in or touching it. This is especially dangerous when someone eats a food they did not know they were allergic to and is unprepared for the anaphylactic reaction.

Lifesaving Epinephrine

Epinephrine, also known as adrenaline, is the most effective drug for combating severe allergic reactions. It is a hormone produced naturally by the body, and it can also be produced synthetically (made in a laboratory). When it is injected into an individual at the onset of anaphylactic shock, it produces several changes in the body that can save the person's life. These include raising blood pressure and opening up a throat that has swollen shut to allow for easier breathing. Epinephrine is often prescribed to individuals with severe allergies to food and other substances.

Medical device manufacturers have developed a variety of syringe-type devices for injecting epinephrine into the bodies of people with severe allergies. These devices are easy to use and are similar in appearance to a pen. They deliver medicine immediately into the bloodstream so it can provide relief right away. Users of epinephrine auto-injectors are typically instructed to make injections into the thigh area. There are many different epinephrine auto-injectors on the market. The best known is EpiPen, but in 2017, the company that makes this product increased the price of a two-pack of EpiPen from $90 to $600, making it difficult for the average person to afford and putting people with allergies in the dangerous position of having to choose whether or not to purchase the medicine that could save their life. According to CNBC, "Most EpiPen customers have some form of insurance that covers all or part of the cost of their purchase … But a small fraction of all consumers pay the list price for the device, either because they have no insurance, or because they are buying multiple packs of EpiPens and only one pack is covered by their health plan."[7]

A more affordable alternative is Adrenaclick, which is sold through the drugstore chain CVS. The store made a deal with the Adrenaclick manufacturer to drop the price of a two-pack from $300 to $110. The manufacturer also offered a $100 coupon, making the price only $10. People who have a prescription for epinephrine can buy up to three two-packs at this price from CVS. If they do not live near a CVS, they can still use the coupon at other pharmacies. With health insurance, that may cover the total cost of the two-pack; without insurance, according to *Consumer Reports* magazine, the final price would be about $100. Although this is expensive, it is far more affordable than the EpiPen and, for some people, could make the difference between life and death.

People with food allergies try their hardest to avoid their allergens, but sometimes they unknowingly eat something that contains one of those foods. That is why doctors urge people with severe food allergies to keep their auto-injectors with them at all times, stored in a way that protects them from extreme heat or cold. In addition, family members, teachers, friends, and parents of friends should all become familiar with auto-injectors and learn how to use them in case the person with allergies goes into shock and is unable to do it themselves.

Many people with severe food allergies say that epinephrine auto-injectors have enabled them to lead much more "normal" lives than would otherwise be possible. Journalist Elizabeth Landau wrote about her auto-injector device, "We've had nearly every meal together for the past 14 years. We've been kayaking on the California coast. We've ridden airplanes, boats, horses, bikes, and an Israeli camel together … The allergy injector has both the dependable and nagging qualities of a

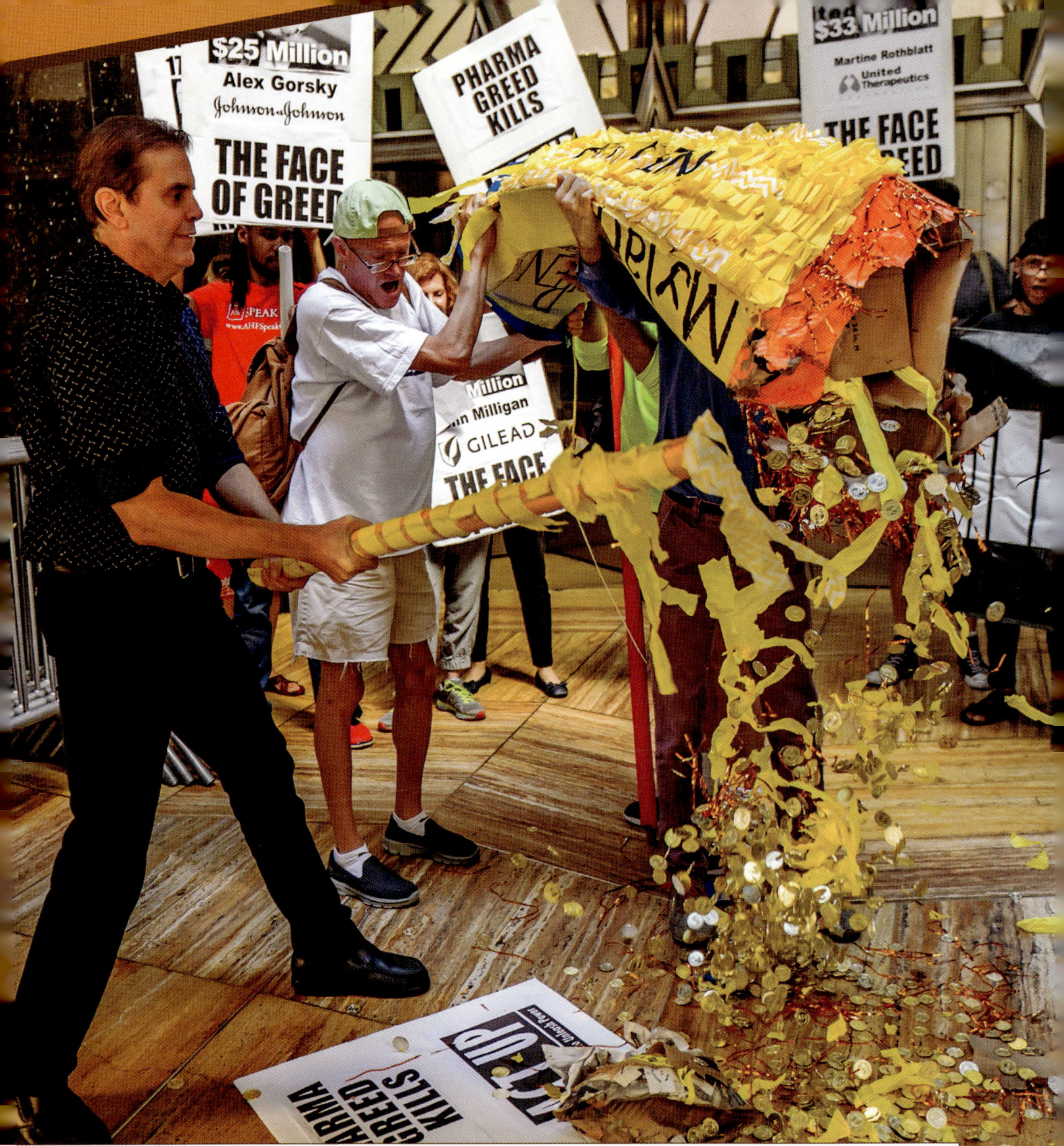

Many people were outraged by the huge increase in the price of EpiPen. Shown here is a protest that took place in 2016 outside the headquarters of Mylan, the maker of EpiPen, in which people smashed a piñata that was made to look like an EpiPen and filled with gold coins to symbolize the pharmaceutical industry's greediness.

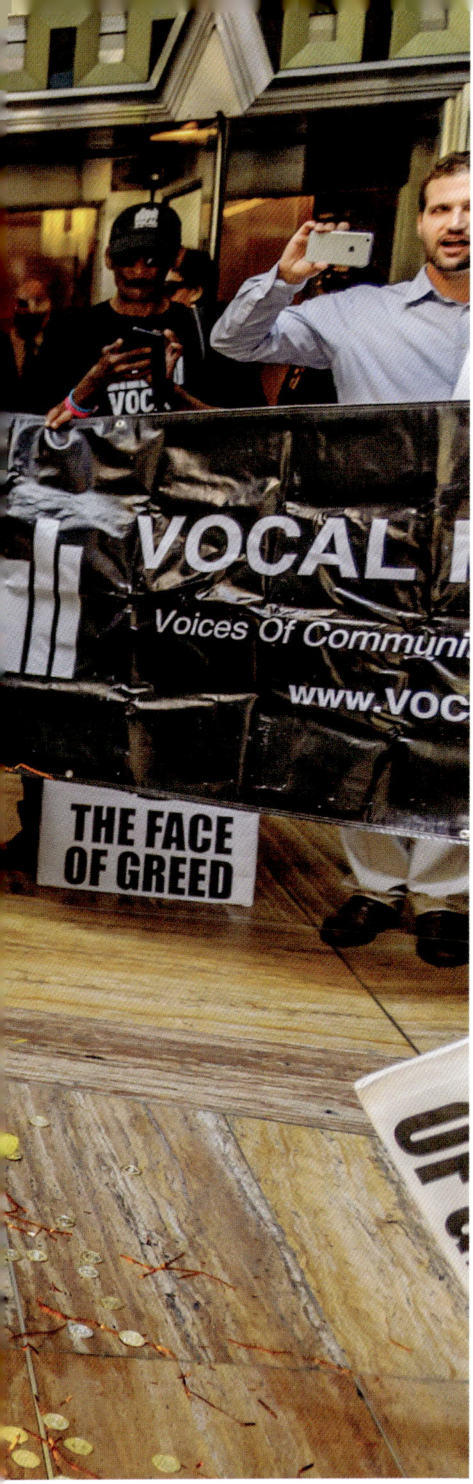

protective older sibling. It promises to be there when I need it, but also has to follow me around to make sure I'm OK."[8]

Allergists emphasize, though, that even after the epinephrine has been injected, people with severe allergic reactions still need to call 911 or quickly get to an emergency room. Qualified medical personnel need to make sure the allergic reaction is under control and does not require further medical intervention.

In addition to carrying epinephrine at all times, people with severe allergies should also wear an allergy alert bracelet or necklace at all times. These tags contain information that can help responders provide proper treatment to people who become too ill to explain their condition. Allergy alert products typically include a list of the person's known allergies and the name and telephone number of an emergency contact person. Some of these items also include additional information, such as personal medical history, health care provider, and additional emergency contact alternatives.

Common Allergy Triggers

While more than 160 different foods are capable of causing allergic reactions, more than half of all reactions in the United States are caused by eight foods: milk, peanuts, eggs, wheat, soy, fish, shellfish (such as shrimp, crab, and clams), and tree nuts (including almonds, hazelnuts, and walnuts).

It is relatively easy for people who are allergic to these foods to avoid eating or drinking these items in their simplest form. People with milk allergies abstain from drinking milk; people who are allergic to eggs stay away from scrambled eggs or omelets at breakfast time; and people who are allergic to tree nuts decline offers of pecan pie. Avoiding these

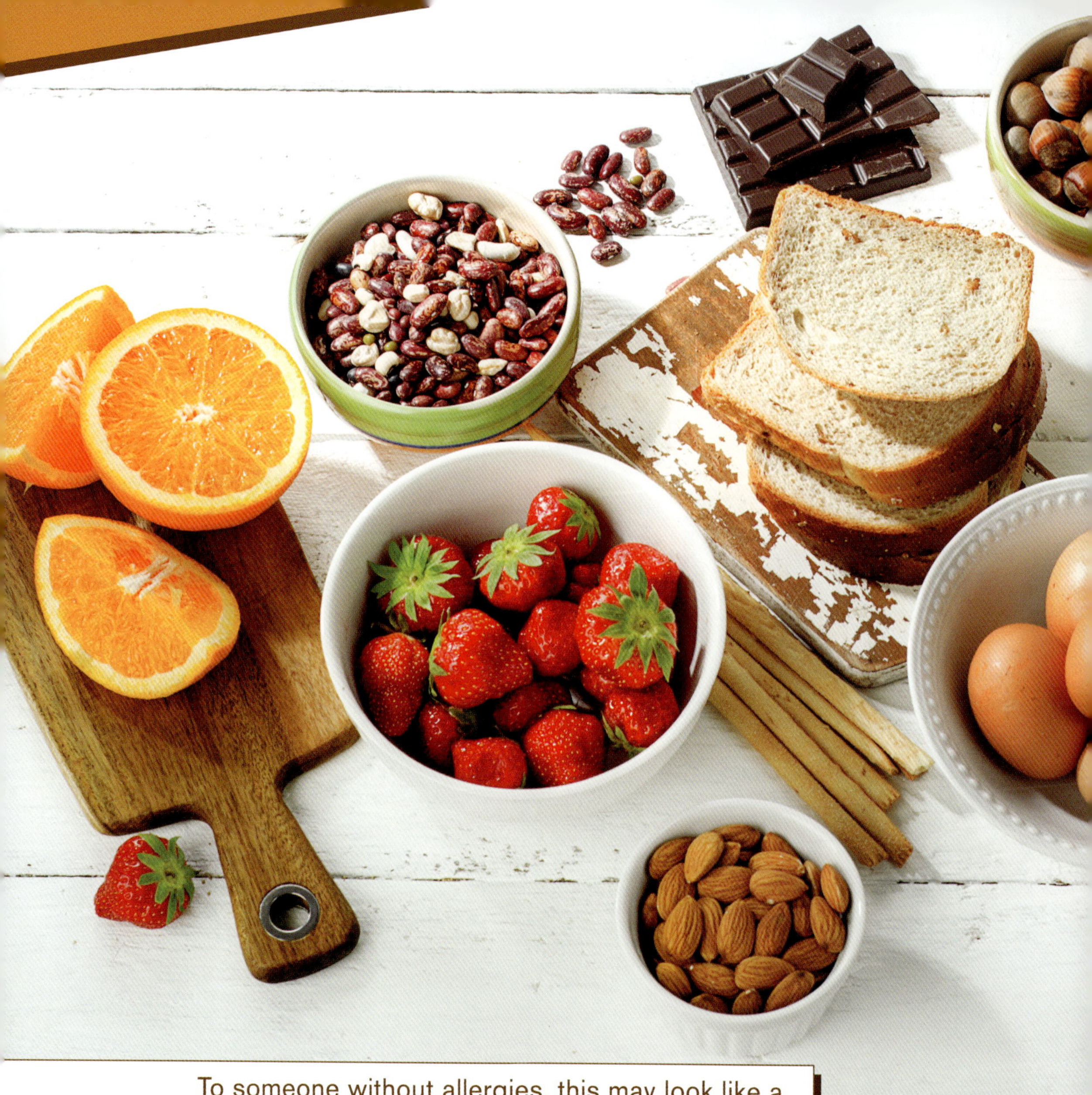

To someone without allergies, this may look like a delicious snack buffet. However, for someone with certain allergies, it can seem like a minefield.

foods completely is tricky, though, because so many of them are hidden as ingredients in other food products. This forces people who have food allergies or who are cooking for someone with an allergy to act as detectives whenever they go to the supermarket or eat at a restaurant. They have to check food labels closely and ask the restaurant staff detailed

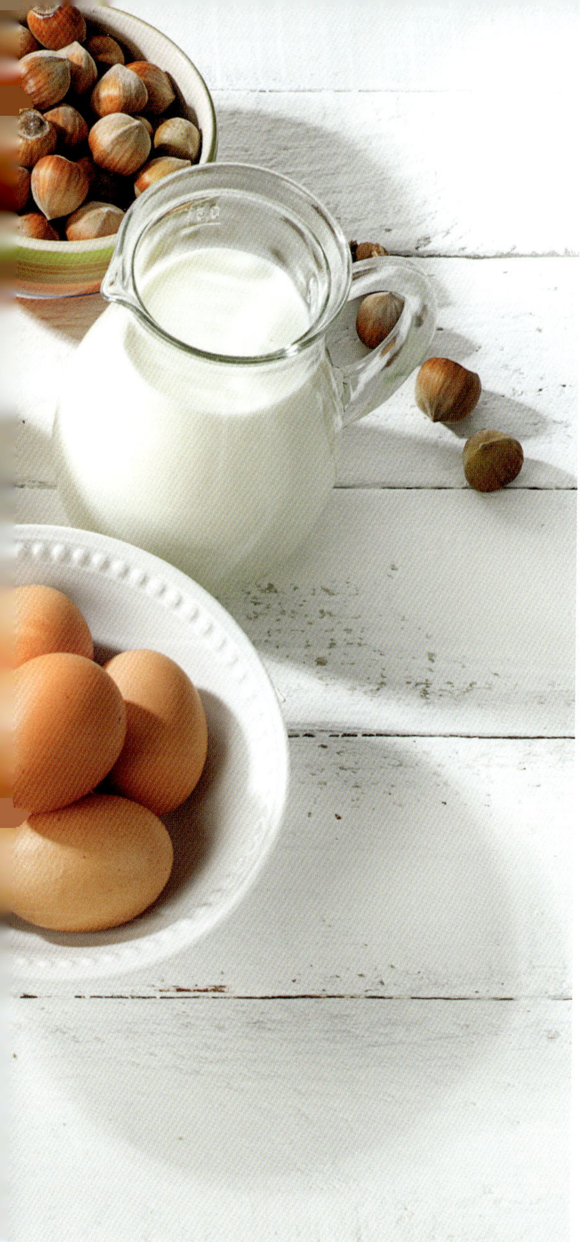

Celiac Disease

Wheat allergies are sometimes confused with celiac disease, which is an ailment of the digestive system. Celiac disease is an autoimmune disorder that causes a negative digestive system reaction to gluten, a group of proteins that are found not only in wheat, but also in other grains such as rye, barley, and oats. This negative response centers on the small intestine, which gradually loses its ability to absorb vitamins and other nutrients. People with celiac disease thus run a higher risk of developing medical conditions such as malnutrition, anemia (a shortage of healthy red blood cells), or osteoporosis (loss of bone density). In contrast, a wheat allergy is an immune system's response to wheat, not just to gluten. Someone who has only a wheat allergy can still eat other grains with gluten in them. It also does not cause the same damage to the digestive system that celiac disease does. An autoimmune disease attacks healthy body cells, causing damage to tissues and organs; an allergy attacks the perceived invader—in this case, wheat.

questions to make sure the food they are purchasing is not contaminated with any of their allergens.

Dangerous Ingredients

It can be hard for someone to get used to eating in a way that will not trigger their allergies, especially if they are allergic to a food they love. Additionally, depending on what food item the person is allergic to, the number of foods they can eat may decrease dramatically. For example, cow's milk is used not only to make popular foods such as cheese, butter, and ice cream, it is also an ingredient in a "multitude of foods, from baby foods to breads to baked goods and milk chocolate, as well as all kinds of processed foods, so avoiding milk typically involves scratching about half of the most common foods off your grocery list. The good news is that the food industry offers plenty of milk, cheese, butter, ice cream, and yogurt substitutes."[9]

It can be difficult for people to identify food allergens because sometimes they do not think to check the ingredients for it. Certain allergens can be in things no one would imagine—including some things that are not even food. For example, peanut oil has been used in products such as hamster feed, lotion, and shampoo. Someone with a severe allergy should avoid these products even though they are not eating them because absorbing them through the skin may still cause a reaction.

In food products, peanuts and tree nuts (such as walnuts, almonds, and pistachios) are sometimes present in a wide assortment of baked goods, including breads, cakes, and pastries. They also are commonly found in various breakfast bars, cereals, chocolate bars and other candies, and ice cream products. Asian foods and vegetarian menus rely heavily on peanuts and other nuts as well. They are used as ingredients in certain salad dressings and condiments, such as barbecue sauce. It is crucial for people who face this issue to proceed carefully—especially in cafeterias and restaurants where strangers are preparing their food.

A Closer Look

According to the Asthma and Allergy Association of America, more than 15 million people in the United States suffer from allergic asthma, or asthma that is set off by an allergen. Allergic asthma is the most common type of asthma.

Eggs are traditionally a major ingredient in cakes, cookies, doughnuts, muffins, pancakes, pretzels, waffles, and other baked goods. They

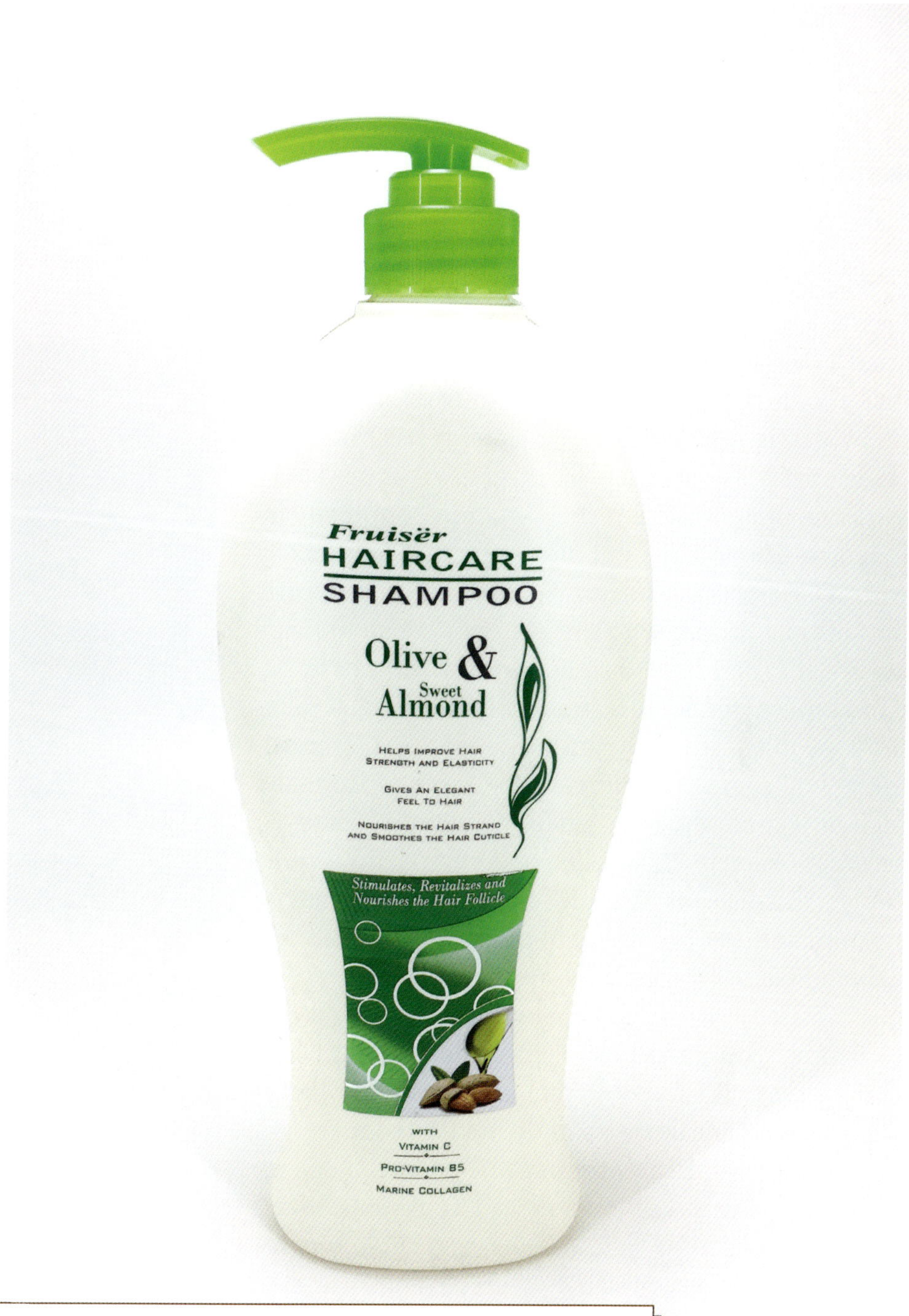

Almond oil is a common ingredient in beauty products such as shampoos and lotions.

also may appear in a wide range of other foods, including candy bars, certain coffee beverages, chicken strips and other breaded meats, eggnog, ice cream, icing, marshmallows, mayonnaise, meatballs and meatloaf, pasta, pudding, salad dressings, sauces, sherbet, and soups. Some food items are made with egg substitutes, but allergic buyers should beware, because these foods often just remove the yolk and still contain egg whites.

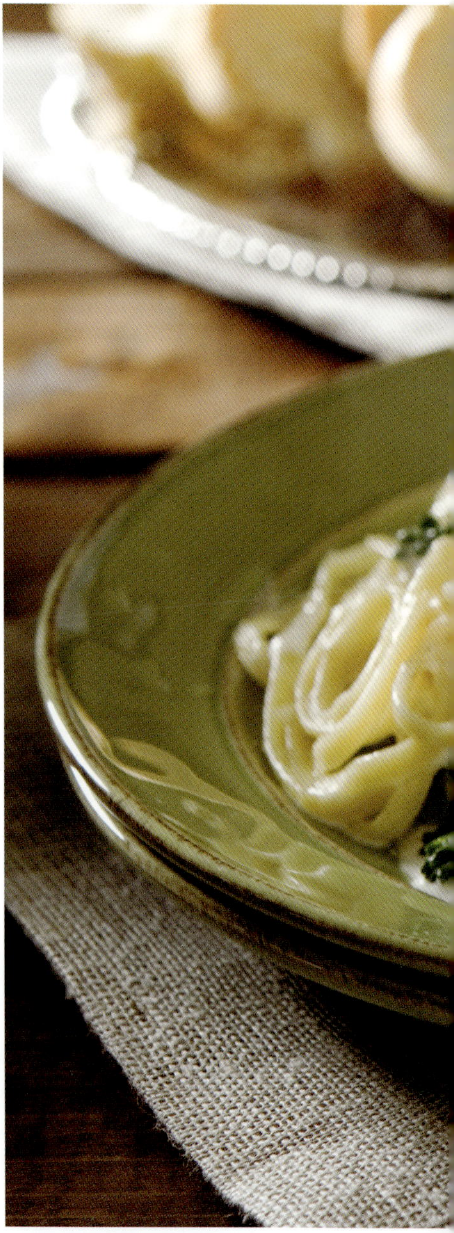

Fish and shellfish allergens are among the easiest to avoid because they are not mixed into many other foods. Nonetheless, there are a few food items that should be approached carefully. One is gelatin, which is sometimes made using fish. Others include Caesar salads, some brands of barbeque sauce, Worcestershire sauce, the vitamin supplement Emergen-C, calcium supplements that are made with oyster shells, and some pet foods. It is worth noting that people who are allergic to fish are not always allergic to shellfish and vice versa. There are two families of shellfish: mollusks and crustaceans. Most people with a shellfish allergy are allergic to both, but some are allergic to just one. Mollusks include clams, mussels, snails (generally listed as escargot on menus), whelks, and even octopus and squid. Crustaceans include crab, lobster, prawns, shrimp, and sea urchins. Food labeling laws in the United States only require crustacean ingredients to be pointed out with an allergy warning on packages, so people with a mollusk allergy should familiarize themselves with the different words for mollusks and carefully check the ingredients for them.

Soybeans and soy products are found in sauces and soups of various kinds, as well as in some baked goods, canned tuna fish, cereals, crackers, and infant formula. Soy is related to green beans, lentils, peanuts, peas, and other legumes, and people who are allergic to one of these foods are often allergic to one or more of the others as well.

Wheat proteins are often hidden in sauces that have multiple ingredients, such as soy sauce, or deep-fried foods that may be cooked with other foods containing wheat. Other food items that come from wheat include bread crumbs, bulgur, cereal extract, club wheat, couscous, durum, einkorn, emmer, farina, flour, hydrolyzed wheat protein, Kamut,

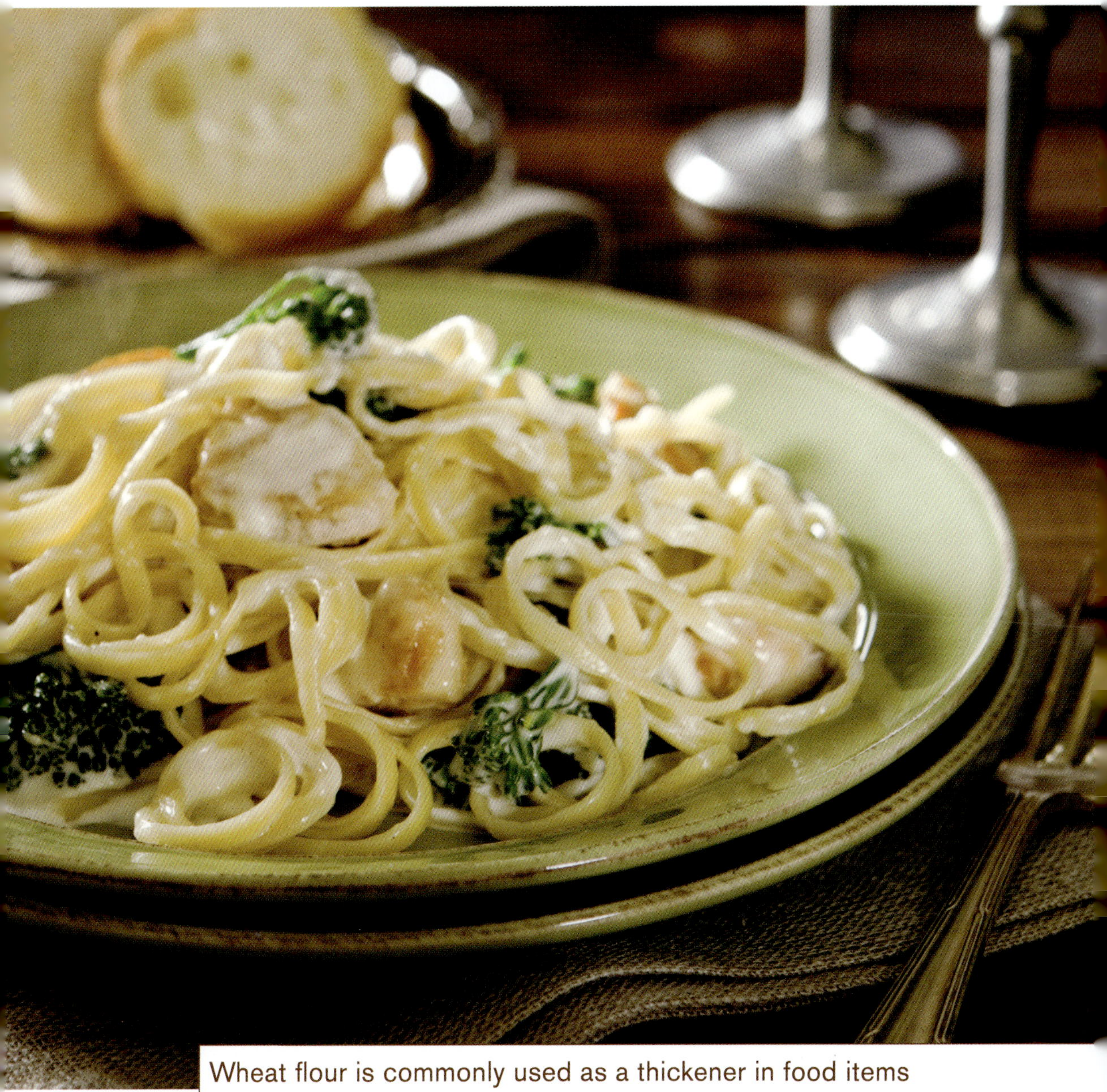

Wheat flour is commonly used as a thickener in food items that do not otherwise contain wheat, such as some sauces.

matzoh, pasta, seitan, semolina, spelt, sprouted wheat, triticale, wheat germ oil, and wheatgrass.

In some cases, young people with food allergies can "outgrow" them over the years. According to the American Academy of Allergy, Asthma & Immunology (AAAAI), 80 percent of children are likely to outgrow an allergy to milk by the time they turn 16. A similar number will eventually outgrow an allergy to eggs, and even more will outgrow an allergy to wheat or soy. Unfortunately, allergies to peanuts and tree nuts are the most likely to remain for life.

Chapter Two

FOOD ALLERGIES ON THE RISE

There is no denying that having a food allergy complicates life. It can seem unfair that while one person can eat anything they want, another has to worry about everything they put in their mouth. This is hard not only on children with food allergies, but also on those who take care of them. A diagnosis of a food allergy can cause an entire household to adopt new ways of eating.

Researchers say that the number of children with severe allergies is on the rise. Allergies to things in the wider environment—especially certain foods—have increased dramatically across the United States over the past 50 years. Scholars estimate that in 1950, less than 15 percent of the total U.S. population had allergies of one type or another. Today, the AAAAI and other research organizations frequently put that number above 50 percent.

More Allergies and Worse Reactions

A big part of this increase in allergies is an increase in food allergies specifically. Not only is the number of reported allergic reactions rising, people with food allergies are also experiencing more severe reactions when exposed to allergens. "Allergists say they're now seeing more children with multiple allergies than ever before, not just to 1950s staples such as milk and wheat—but to global foods we have adopted since, like sesame and kiwi," wrote journalist Claudia Kalb in 2007. "And allergies many kids outgrow—like those to eggs—seem to be lingering longer than they did in the past."[10]

Scientists and doctors can point to a wide range of supporting studies when they declare that food allergies are getting worse. According

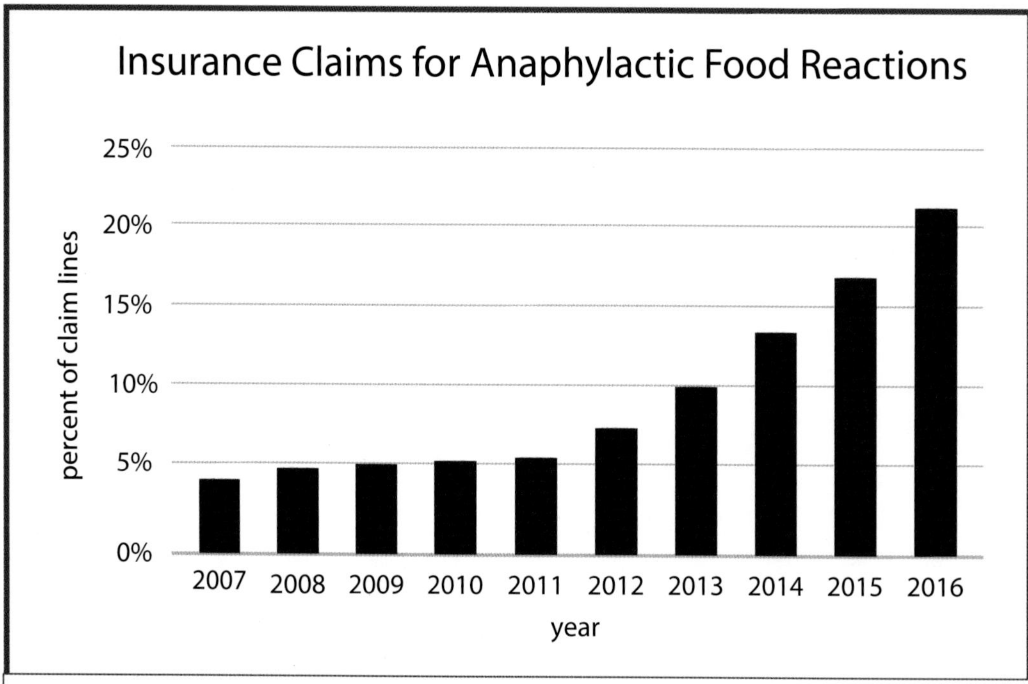

In 2017, a nonprofit organization called FAIR Health released a study about allergies. It showed that the number of insurance claims people had made for anaphylactic reactions had risen dramatically between 2007 and 2016.

to a 2013 report from the Centers for Disease Control and Prevention (CDC), food allergies among children rose by approximately 50 percent between 1997 and 2011. A study from the Mount Sinai School of Medicine published in 2010 stated that the childhood allergy rate for peanuts alone more than tripled between 1997 and 2008. It is also estimated that nearly 6 million school-aged children across the United States now have some type of food allergy.

Deaths and hospitalizations from severe reactions to food allergens are on the rise as well. A long-term study conducted by the Mayo Clinic in Minnesota found that the number of anaphylaxis cases in the United States that were triggered by food allergies increased from 21,000 per year in 1999 to 51,000 per year in 2008.

Allergists admit that it can be difficult to determine exactly how many people have food allergies. In November 2018, *Pediatrics* magazine published a study indicating that nearly 8 percent of American kids have at least one food allergy and that 20 percent of them had visited an emergency room for an allergic reaction in the previous year. The study also found that 41 percent of those diagnosed have a prescription for an epinephrine auto-injector.

A Closer Look

According to a 2019 article by *Forbes* magzine, 200,000 people in the United States seek emergency treatment for food allergies every year.

Food allergy symptoms can closely mirror the symptoms of a cold or the flu. Dr. Hugh Sampson, who is the director of the Jaffe Food Allergy Institute at Mount Sinai Medical Center, explained why this is such a problem. "It's always tempting to relate some physical event or symptom back to what you've put in your mouth," he said. "Hypochondria is a big problem in [tracking food allergies]."[11] Hypochondria describes a situation in which someone mistakenly believes they are sick or attributes their illness to the wrong cause. People with food allergies, according to Sampson, are more likely to believe that a contagious illness is actually an allergic reaction. Someone may think, "There must have been an allergen in the food I ate last night," rather than thinking that they caught the cold that is going around. This can make it difficult for someone to accurately track the instances of their allergic reactions and can lead to people unnecessarily avoiding certain foods.

There are several leading theories about the root causes of the recent increase in food allergies. Some people believe that it can be attributed to new chemical additives in food. Others think it is due at least partially to an increased emphasis on hand washing and other changes in sanitary practices. Heredity and the timing of children's first introductions to food have also been mentioned as possible factors. However, some people believe food allergies have not increased that much, but rather are just being diagnosed more often.

The Role of the Food Industry

Industrial farming and modern food processing are increasingly suspected as factors in the rise of food allergy rates. While the use of

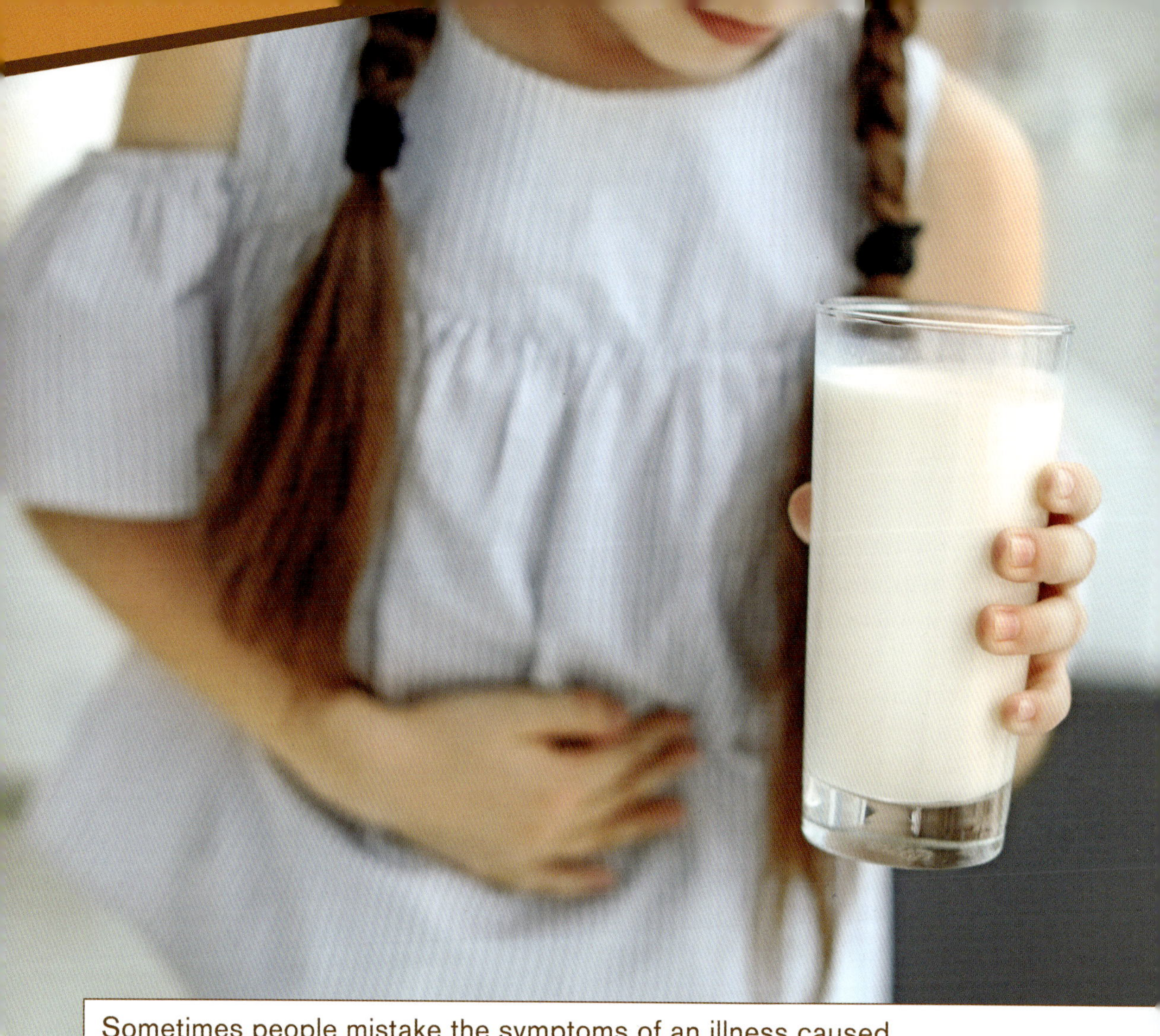

Sometimes people mistake the symptoms of an illness caused by a virus or bacterium for the symptoms of an allergic reaction.

fertilizers and insecticides increases the amount of food that can be grown, these chemicals can remain on crops after they enter the marketplace. Livestock has increasingly been raised on growth hormones to increase both meat and milk production, leading some people to express concern over how those hormones might affect people who ingest those food products. In addition, many prepackaged and processed foods are infused with artificial ingredients to enhance flavor and extend shelf life. Relatively few studies have been done to measure the effects of such practices on human health.

The food industry insists that all the chemicals it uses are safe, and companies point out that their production methods enable them to offer huge quantities of good-tasting food to American consumers at generally low prices. The U.S. Food and Drug Administration (FDA) has approved all the chemicals used in processed food, and many people believe this is proof that they are safe to eat. In 2015, the organization Sense About Science (SAS) stated that the true problem is not the food but the misinformation surrounding allergies, such as the idea that an intolerance and an allergy are the same thing. In an article for the British newspaper the *Guardian*, SAS director Tracey Brown said confusion between allergies and intolerances and misdiagnosis of allergies were "the biggest mess for science communication, where myths, misinterpreted studies and quackery [fake medicine] collide with under- and over-diagnosis ... The costs are huge—unnecessary actions for some and not enough action for those whose lives depend on it."[12]

However, others disagree, fearing that not enough research has been done to show what the long-term effects of these chemicals might be. Many scientists, doctors, and consumers believe that industrial food production has resulted in an increase in outbreaks of foodborne illness—sickness from germs that get passed through food. Some observers also express concern that the chemicals added to food might be contributing to public health problems ranging from early puberty to higher rates of cancer. With all of these concerns, it seems natural to some people that processed food could also be responsible for higher rates of allergies. "Modern food processing," explained *Science News*, "alters natural proteins and adds nonfood substances never before consumed in large amounts."[13]

Critics believe that the government agencies that oversee the safety of the food supply, such as the FDA, should pay more attention to the role that food additives could be playing in rising rates of food allergies and other public health problems. "It is entirely possible that the cumulative effect of eating like this over a generation or so has caused more people to become sensitive to food," wrote Eliza Meyer, who raised two children with food allergies. "While the FDA releases its umpteenth report on the dangers of fat in the American diet, consider that everyone might be missing the point entirely. What difference does fat make when your body is being forced to digest chemicals it was never intended to?"[14]

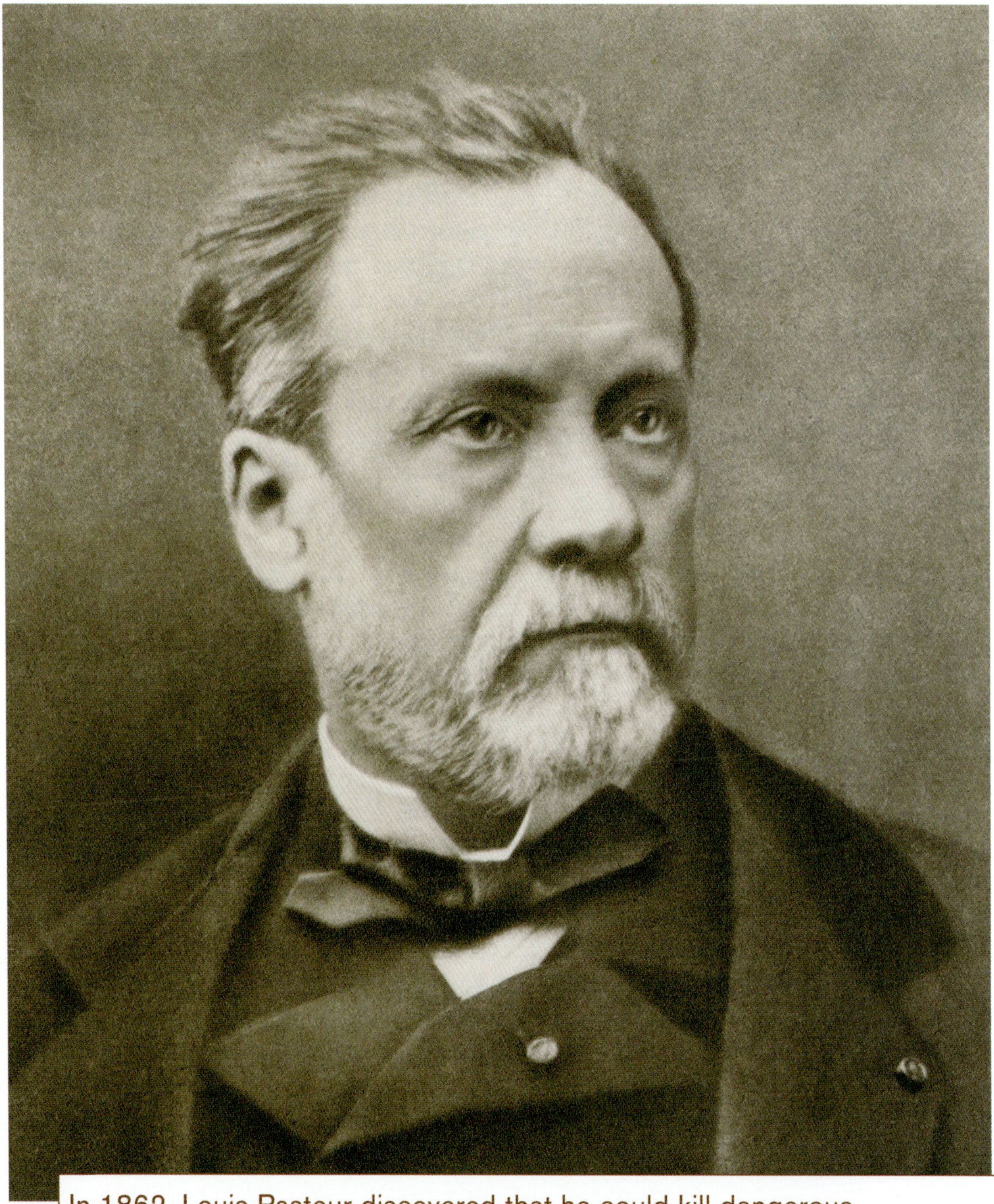

In 1862, Louis Pasteur discovered that he could kill dangerous bacteria in milk through a process of heating and cooling. This technique was called pasteurization after him, and today, nearly all dairy products that are sold in the United States are pasteurized.

Writer Joanna Blythman expressed a similar sentiment, saying, "Ask any older person you know whether they remember anyone with a food allergy back in their day. The answer will almost invariably be no … Our food is now made in qualitatively different ways … Almost all the milk we drink goes through the high pressure and heat of homogenisation and pasteurisation. And the result? It's not the same … and it may not be so digestible as a result."[15] However, as SAS pointed out, myths such as these can cause unnecessary distress and do not account for how modern food processing has helped people. In addition to providing more food cheaply, some changes in manufacturing have to do with safety. Pasteurization, for instance—the process of heating milk to kill germs—has led to a dramatic decrease in illnesses and deaths caused by drinking milk or eating cheese made with raw milk. People with lactose intolerance, or a sensitivity to dairy, lack an enzyme called lactase that processes the chemical lactose that is found in milk. Some people believe the heating process of pasteurization damages the lactase enzyme in milk and makes it more difficult for people to digest, but the FDA and other scientific groups have noted that this is a myth: Pasteurization does not affect a person's reaction to milk because neither raw nor pasteurized milk contains lactase; it is present only in people's bodies.

Growing Awareness of Allergies

Many researchers have suggested that the apparent rise in the rate of allergies is due to confusion between an intolerance and an allergy. In 2019, *TIME* magazine reported on a study of 40,500 Americans published in the medical journal *JAMA Network Open*. The study found that although 19 percent of adults believe they have a food allergy, only 11 percent of them have allergy symptoms. According to *TIME*,

> *This discrepancy [difference] suggests that quite a few adults are conflating [confusing] allergies with less-severe food intolerances, which typically come with minimal digestion-related symptoms, the researchers write. If someone is truly allergic to a food, eating it can trigger a potentially life-threatening immune response. (People who are lactose intolerant, for example, may experience bloating, stomach pain and gas after eating dairy products, while those with a true milk allergy can experience wheezing, hives and anaphylaxis.)*[16]

The study also found that less than half of the people who said they had an allergy had gotten an official diagnosis from a doctor. According to the study's authors, getting a medical diagnosis "could help true sufferers get the treatment and avoidance tips they need—and spare those with only intolerances from a lifetime of unnecessary precautions."[17]

It is generally accepted that better education and reporting over the last several decades has factored into the increased numbers of those suffering from food allergies. Today's parents, pediatricians, and educators are better informed about the signs of possible reactions to food allergens. Support groups and other resources are readily available online, and the media reports on new medical studies every day. Caregivers today, some experts believe, are simply more likely to recognize an allergic reaction and to seek medical help.

If this theory is true, then research studies may have underestimated how many children and adults suffered from food allergies in earlier times. "A couple of decades ago, it was not uncommon to have kids sick all the time and we just said 'They have a weak stomach' or 'They're sickly,'"[18] explained Anne Muñoz-Furlong, founder of the Food Allergy & Anaphylaxis Network (FAAN), now known as Food Allergy Research & Education (FARE).

A Closer Look

According to the National Institutes of Health (NIH), about 65 percent of the human population is lactose intolerant but not allergic to milk.

According to Muñoz-Furlong and others, today's parents are more aware that food allergies are a possible source of health problems. As a result, they are more likely to take their kids to allergists to see whether food allergies are the source of their stomachaches, rashes, and runny noses. These specialists have also become more likely to pass their findings along to researchers. This combination of factors might cause researchers to draw the conclusion that food allergies are rising when, in reality, it is only reports of food allergies that are rising.

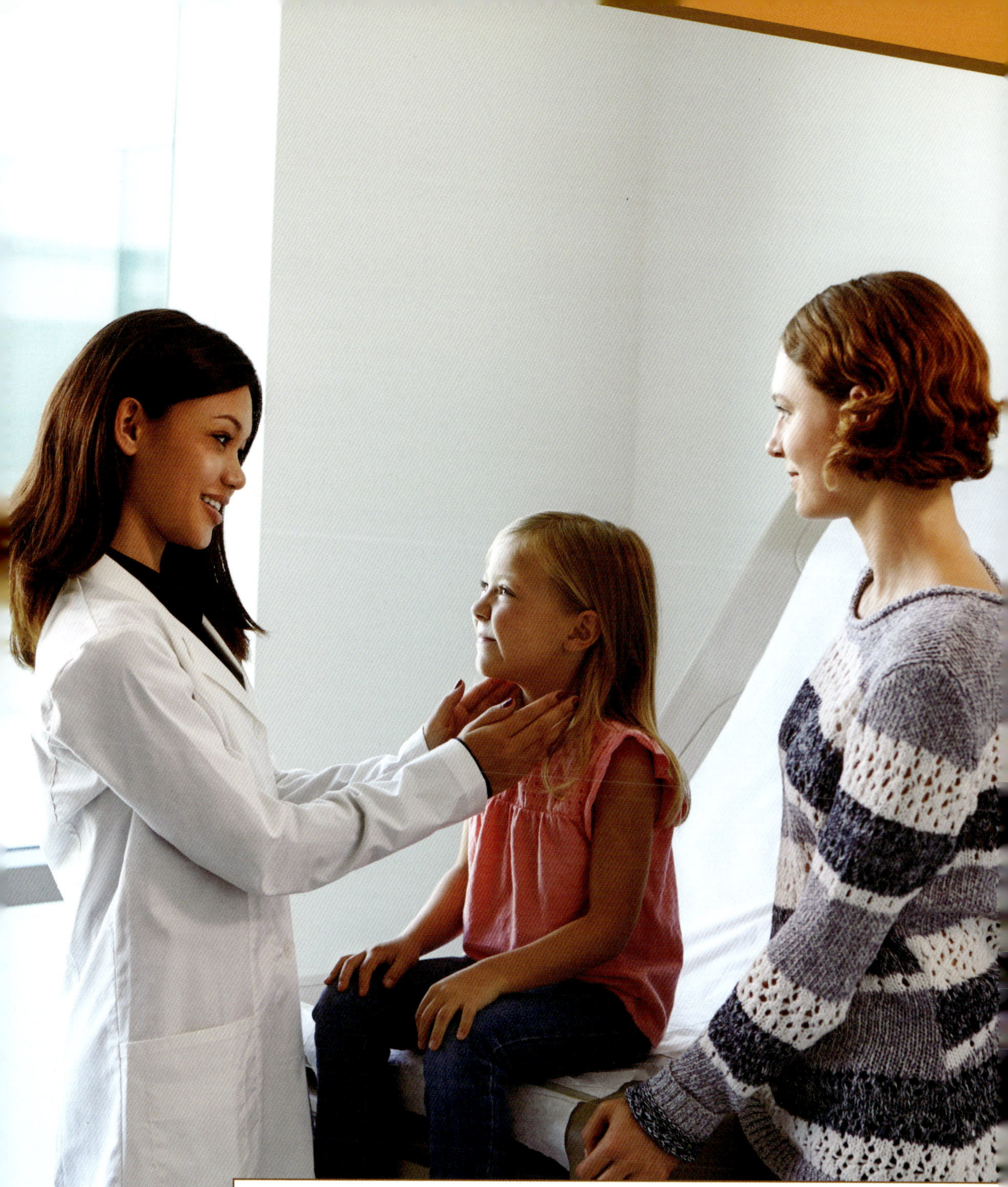

Doctors today are better educated about food allergies than they were in the past.

Too Clean?

While greater awareness of food allergies is almost certainly a factor in the increased rate of food allergy diagnoses, it is unlikely that it is the only factor. One of the most popular theories as to what has caused these increased rates is the hygiene hypothesis. According to supporters of this hypothesis, the immune system is strengthened by exposure to pathogens, or germs. Modern children are increasingly shielded from coming into contact with common germs due to a greater emphasis on personal hygiene. Cleansers are often used to sanitize surfaces people frequently come in contact with, and antibacterial soap is often used in bathroom and kitchen settings.

Some people fear that this emphasis on cleanliness kills not only "bad" germs, but "good" germs as well. They believe that children "are protected too much from dirt, bacteria and other germs. Because of this, our bodies and our immune system do not get the education they require to distinguish friend from foe."[19] According to the hygiene hypothesis, underexposure to germs is a main factor in the development of allergies, as the immune system gets confused and starts to attack foods such as peanuts instead of actual germs.

There is some evidence to support this theory. For example, researchers have learned that children who grow up on farms, where they have constant contact with germ-carrying livestock and associated facilities, are less likely to develop allergies. Studies also indicate that children who attend day care—where many other germ-carrying kids can be found—are less likely to develop allergic reactions to food or other allergens. Researchers have also found that children who are delivered through a Cesarean section, or C-section—where, instead of being pushed out of the body, the baby is pulled out through an incision, or cut, in the mother's torso and uterus—tend to be more likely to develop allergies, as are children who are not breastfed. Dr. Kirtly Jones explained the leading theory: "Now, a baby in the uterus the day before it is born is living in a mostly sterile environment. The passage through the mom's birth canal during a labor allows mom's

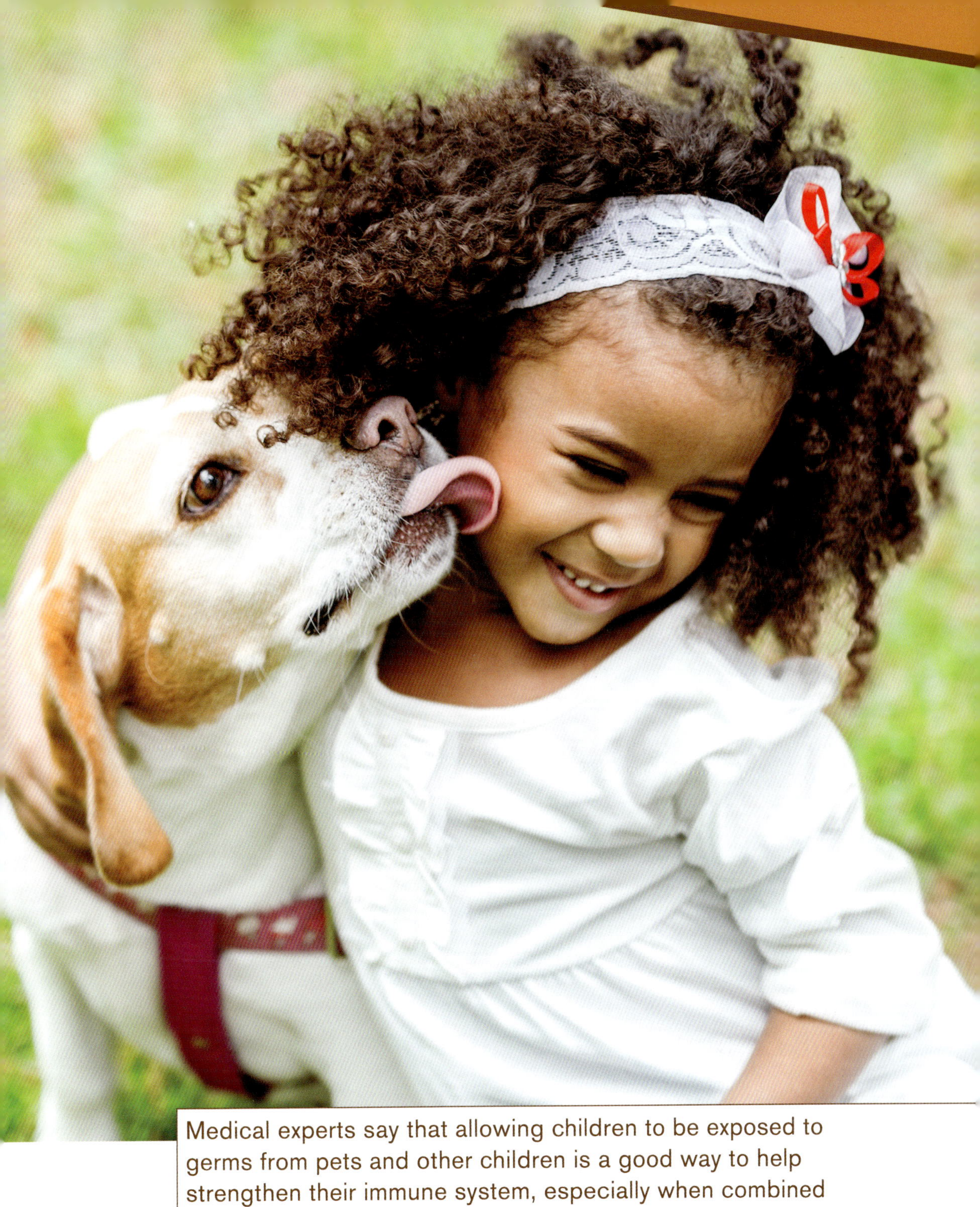

Medical experts say that allowing children to be exposed to germs from pets and other children is a good way to help strengthen their immune system, especially when combined with a decrease in the use of antibiotics and antibacterial soap.

bacteria to colonise the baby, and breastfeeding allows some more."[20] However, Jones noted that the difference between which children get allergies and which do not is small, and having a C-section does not guarantee that someone's child will develop allergies, just as having a natural birth does not guarantee the child will not. Studies are ongoing in this area to try to come to a definitive conclusion.

Some allergists believe that food allergy rates will continue to worsen as society's germ-fighting technologies get even more effective and sophisticated in the years to come. However, microbiologist Tim Yeomans cautioned people against going too far in the opposite direction and rejecting all disease-fighting measures. In an article for the website Allergy Standards, he wrote,

> *The hygiene hypothesis is a possible explanation for this rise [in allergies in developed countries] as we move towards more urbanised [city] living with homes and farms ... now separated to a greater extent. This does not mean that we should ... stop cleaning our homes, invite in farm animals, drink unpasteurized milk or even stop washing ourselves in an effort to educate our immune systems. Importantly sanitation has led to reductions in the cases of typhoid and cholera and other childhood diseases in the developed world.*[21]

The Role of Genetics

Studies show that allergies have a genetic component, meaning that whether someone develops an allergy partially has to do with the genes their parents pass down to them. Genes carry the information in a person's deoxyribonucleic acid (DNA) that plays a role in determining things such as physical traits, personality traits, and the development of certain diseases. The chances of developing a food allergy may be 30 to 50 percent higher for someone who has one parent with a food allergy. If both parents have food allergies, the chances of developing one could be 75 percent higher. Scientists note, however, that specific food allergies are not always passed on from parent to child. Instead, allergenic parents simply pass along genes that put their child at a higher risk for food allergies in general. For example, if a father is allergic to shellfish, his daughter may not be allergic to

The Vaccination Myth

One of the things people fear in regard to the hygiene hypothesis is vaccination. Today, children are given vaccines to immunize them, or protect them from dangerous diseases. Some people believe that by stopping their children from experiencing diseases that were formerly a common part of childhood—such as measles, mumps, and chickenpox—they are not giving the children's immune systems enough work to do, leading to autoimmune diseases and allergies. However, no study has ever proven that vaccines cause allergies. While some studies have noted a link between unvaccinated children and fewer allergies, those studies could not prove whether the cause was vaccines or some other factor—for example, they did not include information on if the children had been delivered by C-section.

According to the website Vaccines Today, the history of Germany provides convincing proof that vaccines have nothing to do with allergies. From 1945 to 1990, Germany was divided into East and West Germany, with different laws in each part. In East Germany, vaccination was required, so nearly 100 percent of children were immunized. East German children also had very low allergy rates. The website went on to explain,

> *After Germany was reunited, vaccination was no longer legally compulsory [required] and the immunisation rate decreased. At the same time, allergies became more common. This would imply that while some aspect (or a combination of aspects) of modern living is responsible for higher allergy rates, vaccination is not part of the equation.*[1]

Rather than making children healthier, numerous studies have shown that choosing not to vaccinate exposes people to far more danger. This is true not only unvaccinated children, but also for people around them. This includes those who cannot be vaccinated because they are too young or allergic to an ingredient in the vaccine, or who are vaccinated but have a disease such as acquired immunodeficiency syndrome (AIDS) that damages their immune system and makes it harder for them to fight off disease.

1. "Do Immunisations Cause Allergies?," Vaccines Today, March 27, 2018. www.vaccinestoday.eu/faq/do-immunisations-cause-allergies/.

shellfish. She is more likely, though, to develop an allergy to another food, such as peanuts or milk, than someone whose father has no food allergies at all. This is why allergy testing is especially important for people whose parents have allergies.

Many Factors to Consider

There may also be cultural factors at work in the development of food allergies. One example of this is the dietary use of peanuts in different parts of the world. In much of Africa and Asia, children are given food containing peanuts at a very young age. Peanut allergies are very rare in these societies. In contrast, physicians in the United States advise limiting or banning peanuts from young children's diets. Meanwhile, the number of children in the United States with peanut allergies continues to rise. Some researchers think that delaying the introduction of a possible allergen to a child's diet may actually put them at a greater risk of eventually developing an allergy to that item.

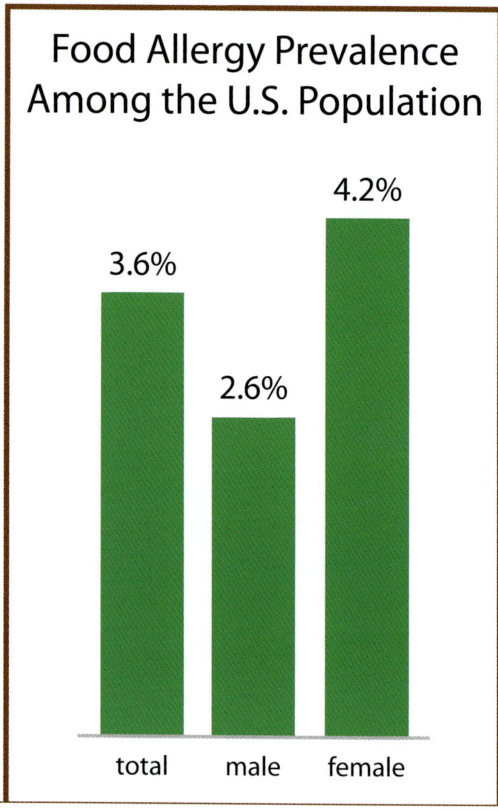

Women are more likely than men to develop food allergies, as this information from *Forbes* magazine shows.

Other environmental factors that have yet to be identified may also play a role. In 2016, Australian news outlet SBS News reported on a study led by Professor Katie Allen of the Murdoch Children's Research Institute in Melbourne, Australia. Allen surveyed 57,000 students in the Australian state of Victoria and found that, although Asian children are genetically predisposed to allergies, they tended not to develop them when they were born in an Asian country, even if they later moved to Australia. In contrast, when Asian children were born in Australia, they had a much higher incidence of food allergies, particularly nut allergies. This study did not answer the question of why this happens, but it provided a starting point for future research. Allen explained, "The risk factors we think are probably important include ... the way the infants are fed food in the first few years of life—and the UV exposure or Vitamin D."[22] Australia is generally much hotter and sunnier than Asia, so increased exposure to the sun could have something to do with the development of allergies, although much more research is needed to discover whether this is true.

Like Allen, other food allergists have concluded that there is not one single culprit responsible for the jump in food allergy rates. They believe that a combination of factors is involved. Further research is necessary to identify all of these various factors to give a better understanding in the future of how people can avoid developing allergies. Until this is better understood, education about diagnosing and treating an allergy is key—not just for the person who has one, but also for family, friends, teachers, food service providers, and more.

Chapter Three

IDENTIFYING A FOOD ALLERGY

The process of diagnosing a food allergy can be frustrating and exhausting. It may take several trips to various doctors and many months of discomfort before being given a preliminary diagnosis. Tests are not always accurate, and some medical professionals may be dismissive. In addition, it is not uncommon for individuals to outgrow an allergy or develop a new one. Fortunately, current tests are more sophisticated than they were in the past, so people have a better chance of having their allergies identified correctly. According to experts, the biggest challenge currently surrounding allergy diagnosis is misinformation about the difference between an allergy and a sensitivity or intolerance, combined with a growing mistrust of the medical industry.

The First Steps Toward a Diagnosis

While it is sometimes very difficult to diagnose a food allergy, other times it is very easy. For example, a severe reaction after consuming almonds would indicate that an individual is allergic to almonds and, therefore, should not eat them. Likewise, less severe reactions can signal an allergy. Experiencing itching, hives, an upset stomach, or increased phlegm production after eating an egg will likely make someone think twice about eating another.

In many other cases, however, the exact nature of the problem can be a little more of a mystery. "Most foods have more than one ingredient," pointed out the KidsHealth website, "so if a kid has shrimp with peanut sauce, what's causing the allergy—the peanut sauce or the shrimp?"[23]

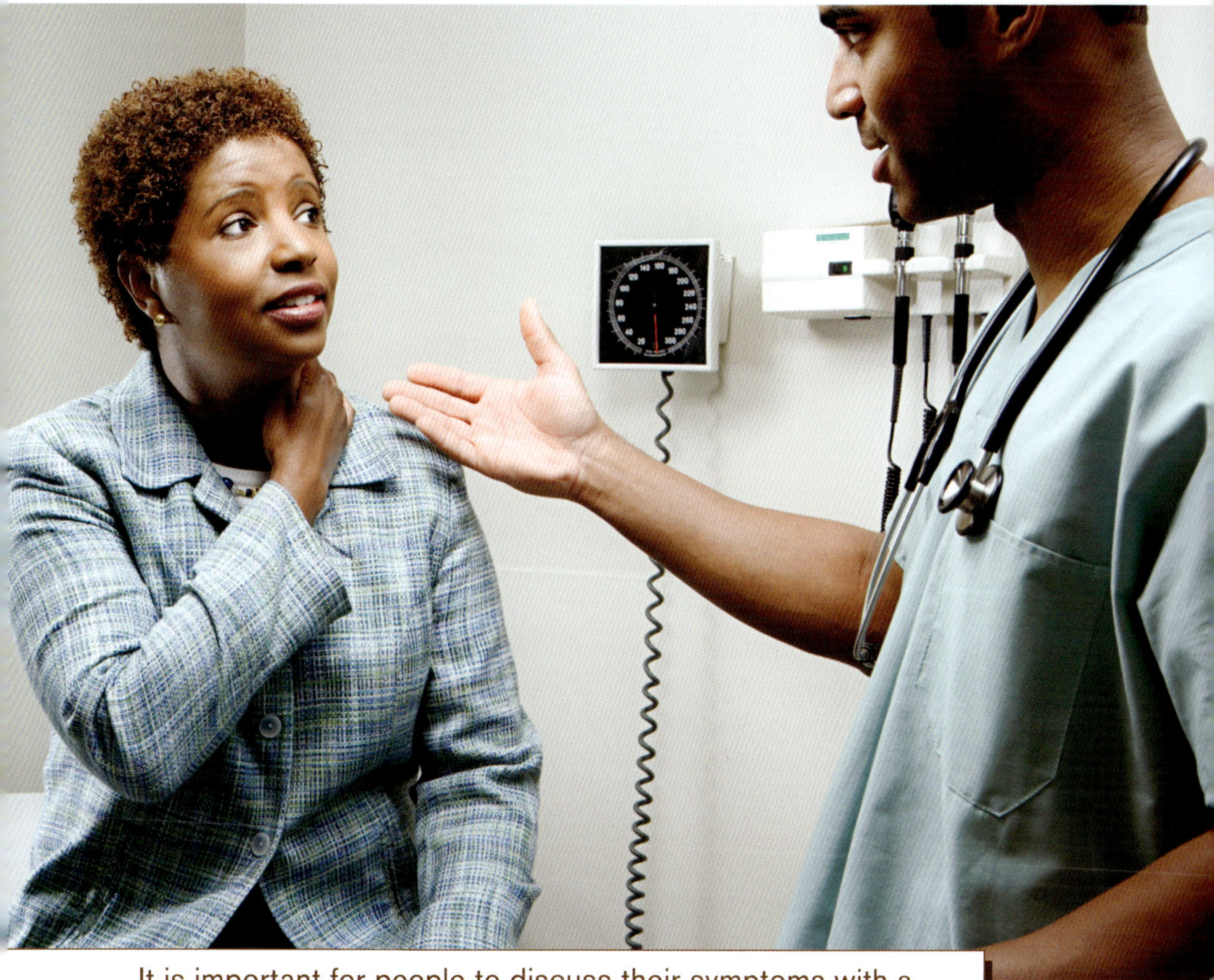

It is important for people to discuss their symptoms with a doctor so they can identify which foods are causing a problem.

While an allergy is an extreme and immediate reaction, a sensitivity has less severe and more delayed symptoms. This makes them harder to diagnose because some of the symptoms do not reveal themselves until 12, 24, or even 48 hours after the food has been consumed. A woman named Joanne explained, “Although my diarrhea occurred soon after I ate foods, my doctor never thought it might be food allergy. He also did not think that my headaches, chest tightness, or joint swelling and stiffness might be delayed reactions to foods. I found it hard to believe that I could react to something that I ate two days ago.”[24]

While the symptoms Joanne experienced were very real and uncomfortable, they indicated that she had a sensitivity or intolerance to certain foods, not an allergy. However, many people are unaware of the difference between these terms and use them interchangeably. According to the AAAAI, "Many people who think they are allergic to a food may actually be intolerant to it. Some of the symptoms of food intolerance and food allergy are similar, but the differences between the two are very important."[25]

A Closer Look

A food intolerance is different than an allergy or a sensitivity. Instead of an immune system response, an intolerance occurs when a person's body lacks an enzyme it needs to break down a certain food. For example, for many East Asian people, the enzyme that helps the body process alcohol is inactive, meaning it is there but does not do what it is supposed to. This leads to an alcohol intolerance.

The lack of knowledge about the difference between an allergy, an intolerance, and a sensitivity can have multiple negative consequences. First, it can lead to a mistrust of doctors. If someone is told by a doctor that they do not have an allergy to a food but they still feel uncomfortable after eating it, they may conclude that the doctor has misdiagnosed them or is not truly listening to them. Second, it can have dangerous consequences for someone with a true allergy. The symptoms of a sensitivity or an intolerance generally occur only after someone has eaten a certain amount of a particular food; if they eat the particular food once in a while, or in very low quantities, then the symptoms may not appear, or they may show up only in mild forms. For this reason, a food server may assume they do not have to be careful about cross contaminating a dish when someone tells them they have an allergy. In contrast to a sensitivity, though, an allergy produces an immediate and sometimes life-threatening reaction when even the smallest amount of a particular food is present in a dish.

Other Allergic Conditions

Although an allergic reaction generally happens immediately, some people have a condition called food protein-induced enterocolitis syndrome (FPIES), which is also known as a delayed food allergy. It is different than a sensitivity because the symptoms it causes—namely, vomiting and diarrhea—are much more severe. In some cases, according to the AAAAI, "symptoms can progress to dehydration and shock brought on by low blood pressure and poor blood circulation. Much like other food allergies, FPIES allergic reactions are triggered by ingesting a food allergen."[1]

Another allergic condition that not all people with allergies experience is called eosinophilic esophagitis (EoE). This condition causes inflammation of the esophagus, which is the tube that sends food from the throat to the stomach. Although the exact cause is unknown, "research suggests that the leading cause of EoE is an allergy or sensitivity to particular proteins found in foods. Most people with EoE have a family history of allergic disorders such as asthma … or food allergy."[2]

1. "Food Allergy Overview," AAAAI, accessed on April 12, 2019. www.aaaai.org/conditions-and-treatments/allergies/food-allergies.

2. "Food Allergy Overview," AAAAI.

Medical professionals have a range of tools at their disposal to determine what kind of food allergies a person might have. Options for diagnosis include skin tests and blood tests, elimination diets, oral food challenges, and detailed surveys of personal and family medical histories. Most allergists turn to some combination of these tools to diagnose exactly what type of food or foods are causing allergy problems for their patients. In addition, some of these same tests can be useful in identifying food intolerances.

Questions and Tests

When attempting to diagnose a possible food allergy, doctors will generally begin by asking an individual about their history of discomfort and illness. Because parents with food allergies are more likely to have

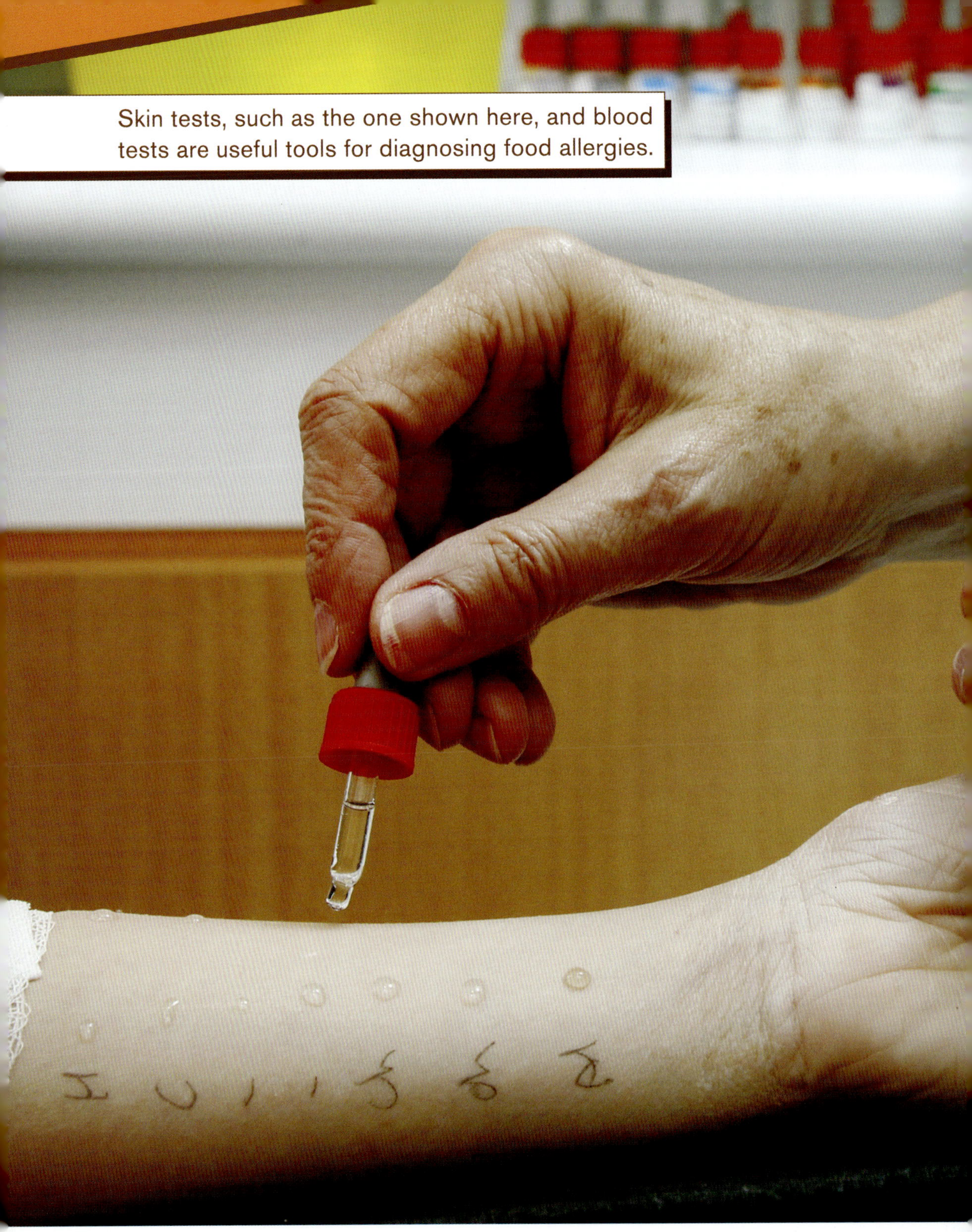

Skin tests, such as the one shown here, and blood tests are useful tools for diagnosing food allergies.

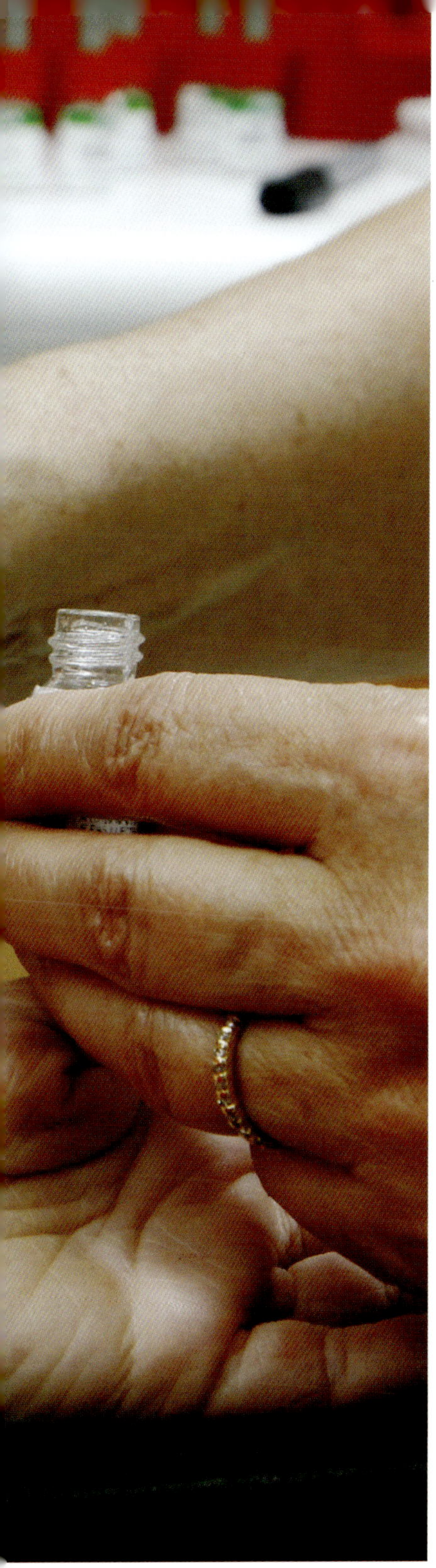

children with some form of food allergy, doctors will also want to know about the health of other family members. Some questions a doctor is likely to ask include:

- What are your symptoms?
- Can you identify particular foods that might be causing these symptoms?
- Has this food caused these symptoms on more than one occasion?
- How much of the food did you eat when the symptoms occurred?
- How was the food cooked or otherwise prepared?
- How long after you consumed the food did your symptoms begin to show?
- How long did the symptoms last?
- Have you ever eaten the suspected food without having any negative health effects?
- Were other potential triggers at work when you ate the food? (Exercise, alcohol, aspirin, and anti-inflammatory drugs can sometimes bring about similar symptoms.)
- Have you ever had these symptoms at a time when you did not consume the suspected food?
- What treatment have you received in the past when these symptoms have appeared?

These questions can help an allergist determine the difference between an allergy, intolerance, sensitivity, and some other medical condition. For example, someone who experiences vomiting and diarrhea once after eating something may only have food poisoning caused by undercooked or tainted food. Once the allergist has this important personal history in hand, they can begin the process of food allergy testing.

A Closer Look

Researchers are unsure exactly why humans developed allergies. One theory is that they originally protected people from eating foods that could be toxic.

Two of the tests most commonly used in diagnosing food allergies are skin prick tests (SPTs) and blood tests. Medical professionals perform an SPT by pricking or scraping a patient's skin with tiny pins coated in a diluted, or weakened, form of the food being tested. While this may sound scary, it is done quickly and with minimal discomfort; it is no more painful than a fingernail scratch. Dozens of foods can be tested in seconds. If an individual is allergic to the food being tested, the skin may turn red or a tiny bump might appear at the site of the application. This indicates an allergic reaction.

If a skin test for a specific food comes up negative, the patient generally does not have to worry about being allergic to that food. Positive tests for food allergies can be misleading, however. Even when an SPT causes hives or another sign of allergies, it does not necessarily mean that the person will have an allergic reaction when eating that food. This phenomenon is known as a false positive. FARE explained the two potential causes of a false positive:

- *When you eat, your digestive system gradually breaks down food proteins into very small pieces. As a result, the allergenic proteins may be so small that the IgE antibodies are unable to detect them, so the food is actually safe for you to eat. But SPTs and blood tests can't mimic the digestive process. Since food proteins are bigger when they interact with your skin or blood, it is easier for the IgE antibodies to "see" the allergens and attack them. This is why your tests may show that you are more sensitive to a suspect food than you really are.*

- *Members of a food "family" often share similar proteins. For example, if you are allergic to peanuts, your tests may show a positive response to other members of the legume family, such as green beans, even if eating green beans has never been a*

> *problem for you. This is known as cross-reactivity. The test is positive because it recognizes a similar protein in peanuts and green beans. But the test hasn't detected the real culprit—another, different protein that is found only in peanuts.*[26]

Allergists also use blood tests to check for food allergies. Blood tests measure the presence of IgE antibodies. Since an SPT gives immediate results, it is the preferred test, but a doctor may order a blood test to confirm the results of the SPT or to get accurate results when a person needs to take an antihistamine (medication that blocks the histamine response). Antihistamines can interfere with the results of an SPT, but not a blood test.

Blood tests have the same potential for false positives as SPTs. In fact, FARE noted that between 50 and 60 percent of tests produce false positives. However, this does not mean that skin and blood tests for food allergies are worthless. For one thing, they almost never produce false negatives, so if the test says someone is not allergic to a certain food, it is virtually certain that they do not have to worry about eating it. This is important for someone who may have a psychosomatic allergy, or one that their mind has convinced their body that they have. These are rare and are generally developed after someone has a bad experience with a certain food—for example, someone who once nearly choked to death on a walnut may find themselves having difficulty breathing the next few times they try to eat something with walnuts in it. This can be mistaken for anaphylaxis, but in reality, it is a panic attack brought on by the memory of their past traumatic experience. If someone believes they have an allergy, they should get tested by a medical professional. If the test turns up negative but they still feel uncomfortable eating that specific food, there is nothing wrong with avoiding it, but they should be sure not to tell people they have an allergy. Instead, they can simply tell people they choose not to eat that food; further explanation is not necessary.

SPTs and blood tests are generally not taken in isolation; someone typically gets them done after they have a negative physical reaction to a certain food. As FARE explained, "if your history suggests that you have had several reactions after eating soy products, and the blood tests show a positive reaction to soy proteins, it is very likely that you do have a soy allergy."[27] Allergists and their patients need to recognize

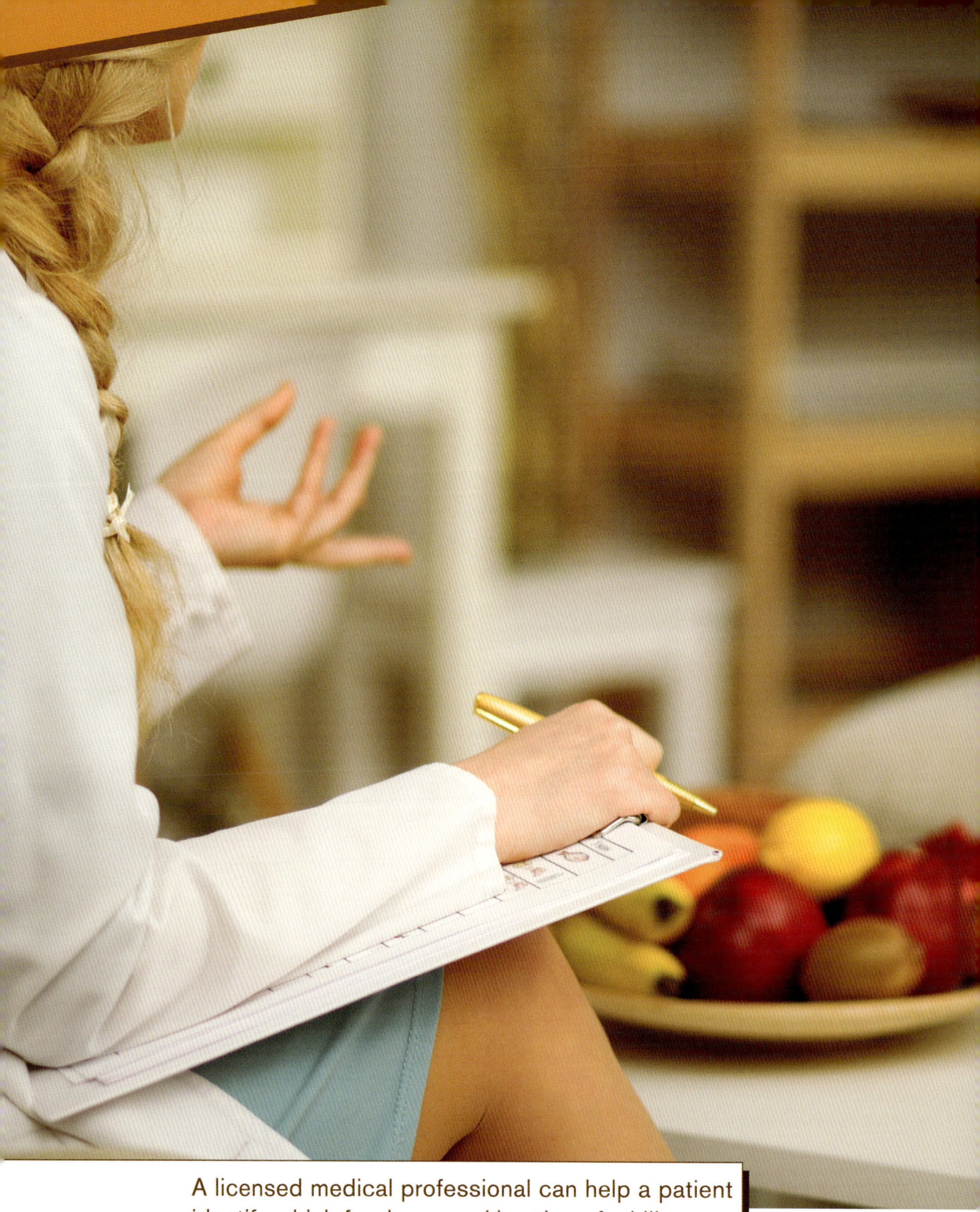

A licensed medical professional can help a patient identify which foods are making them feel ill.

that the results of these tests are more reliable and better understood if other testing procedures are used as well.

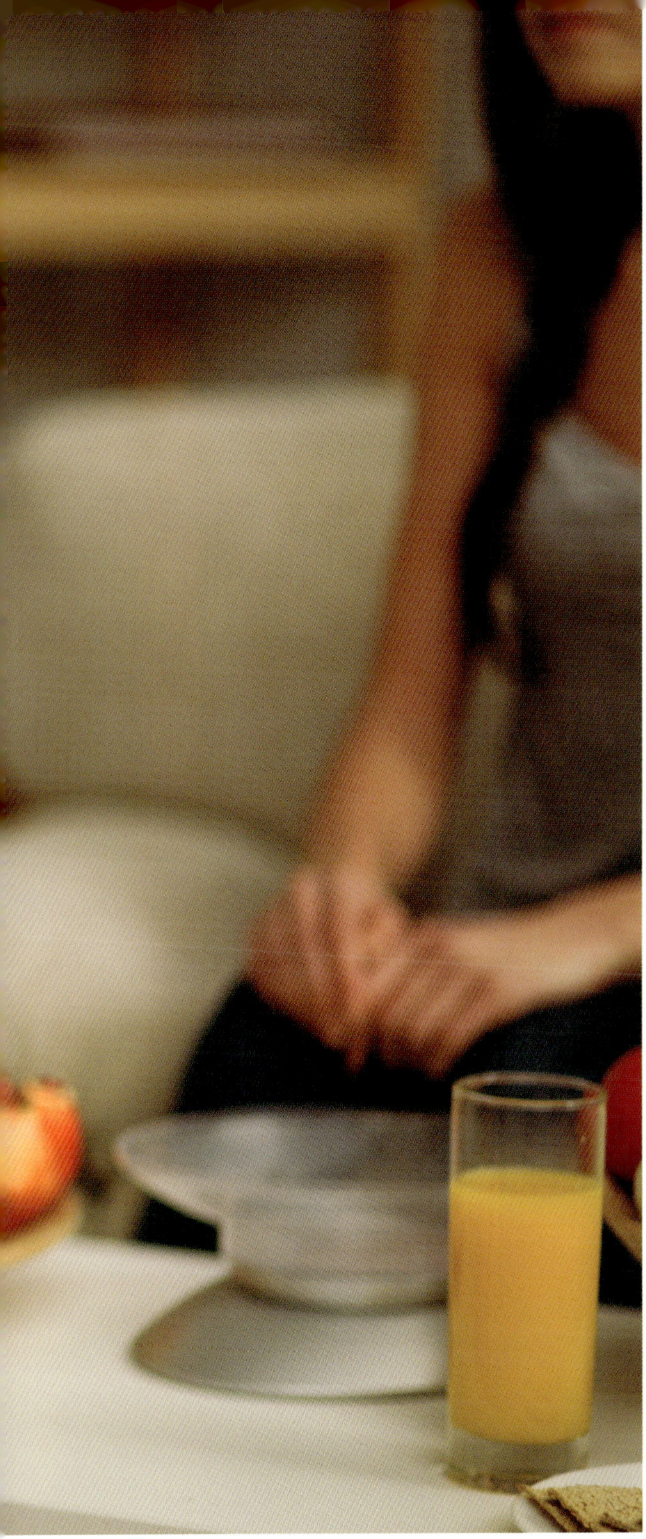

A Useful Tool

Sometimes an elimination diet is used to help test for food allergies. An elimination diet is one in which the most common allergens (and other suspected ones) are totally removed from an individual's diet. After this diet has been followed for several weeks, individual foods are slowly reintroduced to the diet one at a time. For instance, eggs may be reintroduced first. If the individual shows no signs of discomfort after eating them for the first time in weeks, it can be assumed that they are not allergic to eggs. The next day, peanuts might be reintroduced. If there is no sign of a negative reaction, it can be assumed they are not allergic to peanuts. This continues until all foods that were eliminated are reintroduced into the person's diet. The hardest part of an elimination diet is following it faithfully. Consuming even a trace amount of an allergen can ruin the test.

Many allergists and physicians consider elimination diet tests to be a useful tool. They caution, however, that the diets are best used in combination with other allergy detection methods. In addition, people with a

Too Old for Allergies?

Most allergies—including food allergies—first show up during childhood. Sometimes, though, adults can suddenly develop an allergy to foods they have enjoyed all their lives without experiencing any problems. In some cases, a food allergy can develop virtually overnight. "Allergies are like any ailment, they can strike whenever,"[1] said allergist Neeta Ogden. Some people also develop asthma for the first time in adulthood. Cases of adult-onset asthma may or may not be caused by food allergies.

In many cases, the reason why someone suddenly develops an allergy to a food they used to be able to eat is a mystery to scientists. They note, though, that it is a relatively rare phenomenon. According to researchers, an allergy to shellfish is the most frequent type of food allergy that crops up in adulthood. In some rare cases, though, a cause can be identified. For example, in 2017, researchers found that some adults who were suddenly experiencing anaphylaxis for seemingly no reason were actually reacting to a molecule called alpha-gal that occurs naturally in red meat. This rare allergy, which was originally a mystery because it behaves differently than other allergies—for example, symptoms typically appear three to six hours after the person eats red meat, in contrast to other allergies where symptoms can appear within five minutes—developed after the adults were bitten by the Lone Star tick. This type of tick is common in the southeastern United States as well as certain parts of New York, New Jersey, and New England. It is believed that the tick picks up alpha-gal from the animals it bites and transmits it to humans by biting them, causing them to have a reaction when they later encounter alpha-gal in their food and occasionally in other products from mammals, such as wool. More research is necessary to determine exactly why this reaction happens.

1. Quoted in K Aleisha Fetters, "Q&A: Why Do I Suddenly Have Allergies?," *Women's Health*, September 2, 2014. www.womenshealthmag.com/health/a19937829/adult-onset-allergies/.

history of severe allergic food reactions should not be tested through elimination dieting due to the risk that such a reaction may occur when a food is reintroduced. Furthermore, it can be hard to pinpoint food allergies through this method. Some studies indicate that elimination diets remove broad categories of food without sufficient evidence that they cause allergic reactions. "We get patients referred to us all the time who have been placed on very restrictive diets. They may be off ten or twenty foods," said allergist Hugh Sampson. "We go through a full evaluation, and it turns out they are allergic to only one or two."[28] Overly restrictive elimination diets can also make it harder for patients to get the vitamins and nutrients that they need. This is especially true for children, whose food choices are dictated by concerned parents.

Some people believe that oral food challenges are more useful than elimination diets. These are performed with a medical professional

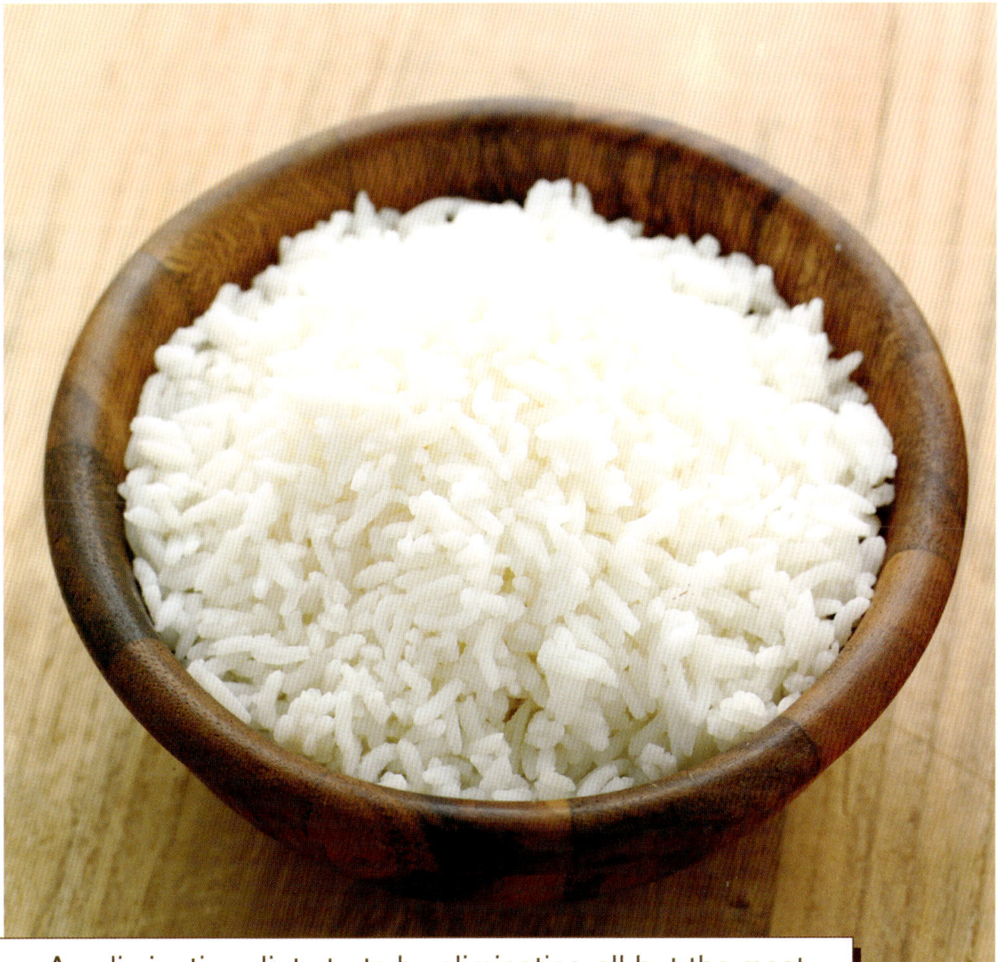

An elimination diet starts by eliminating all but the most basic foods. Some people may eat nothing but rice for the first few days. This is why an elimination diet should not be undertaken unless a doctor considers it necessary.

Too Much Fear

Confusion about food sensitivities versus food allergies and unwillingness to see a medical expert can create a dangerous situation. Some companies sell at-home allergy tests, which are cheaper and faster than a professional allergy test but less reliable. An article in the *Guardian* explained, "The conviction [belief] that a child's chronic lethargy [long-term tiredness] or headaches or eczema is caused by an allergy takes a long time and many tests to prove or disprove. It is tempting to go to an alternative therapist who will do a single test and provide a quick but wrong answer."[1] Many at-home allergy tests claim allergies can cause a long list of symptoms that they are not proven to cause—such as excessive thirst and memory problems—to try to attract more people into buying their product.

Experts say that, among middle-class families, malnutrition—due to parents who put their children on unnecessarily restrictive diets as a result of an inaccurate at-home allergy test—is a bigger threat than food allergies. According to Sense About Science, the at-home tests have no scientific value. One such test is called the Vega test, "which attempts to measure electronic resistance across the skin while the child or adult holds the suspect food in their hand."[2] Other tests involve testing hair samples, but since IgE antibodies cannot be measured through hair, these tests are also useless. Pediatric allergist Adam Fox noted that putting too much faith in these tests can have negative physical and mental effects on children. He said, "There are two challenges. Children need to be given proper diets, but more of it is the unnecessary avoidance of things which aren't harmful, which has a huge impact on the quality of life. A child who can't eat wheat or drink milk can't go to parties."[3] People who suspect they have allergies should always be tested by a medical professional.

1. Sarah Bosely, "Bogus Allergy Tests Causing Real Harm, Say Experts," *Guardian*, June 4, 2015. www.theguardian.com/society/2015/jun/04/bogus-allergy-tests-causing-real-harm-say-experts.

2. Bosely, "Bogus Allergy Tests."

3. Quoted in Bosely, "Bogus Allergy Tests."

present. Very small amounts of suspected allergens are fed to the patient; the medical professional watches as the food is consumed and notes any negative reactions. After a few minutes, a larger amount of the allergen is consumed and reactions to it are recorded. This continues until either the patient consumes a large amount of the suspected allergen and has no reaction—in which case it can be assumed the patient is not allergic—or the patient has a mild reaction.

There are three types of oral food challenge tests. Under an open food challenge test, both the patient and the doctor know which specific food is being tested. Under a single-blind food challenge test, the doctor knows what food the patient is receiving, but the patient does not. The third oral challenge test is the double-blind placebo-controlled food challenge (DBPCFC). This one is the most expensive, but it is also considered to give the most accurate results. In this test, neither the doctor nor the patient knows whether the patient is consuming a suspected food allergen or a harmless substance, which is known as a placebo. This prevents both doctor and patient from misinterpreting any results based on what they expect to see when the patient eats an allergenic food.

An allergist has a very important role in this test. They determine the starting dose for each suspected allergen based on the patient's medical history. The allergist also decides whether to increase the dosage, determines how long each dose should be monitored for delayed reaction, interprets the results of the oral food challenge, and makes dietary recommendations that will keep the patient in good health.

Allergists say that oral food challenges are the most reliable food allergy testing procedures available. Studies seem to confirm this viewpoint. In 2010, for example, the *Journal of Pediatrics* published a study involving a group of Denver, Colorado, schoolchildren who had been classified as food allergic. After these children took oral challenges, they were able to resume eating about 90 percent of the foods that had previously been declared off-limits because of skin tests and blood tests.

Oral food challenges are not without problems: They are expensive, time consuming, and can provoke anxiety among young test takers. However, the tests are very safe. The amount of the suspected allergen a patient starts off eating is tiny, and the dose is increased very gradually. According to FARE, most people have mild reactions, such as hives. The reactions may be unpleasant, but the tests stop long before any life-threatening symptoms occur. This is why oral food challenges are given only by allergy experts and researchers rather than general family doctors: They are the most knowledgeable about how to keep the patient safe during the test. However, because there are fewer allergists than general practitioners, the waiting lists for taking the test are often long.

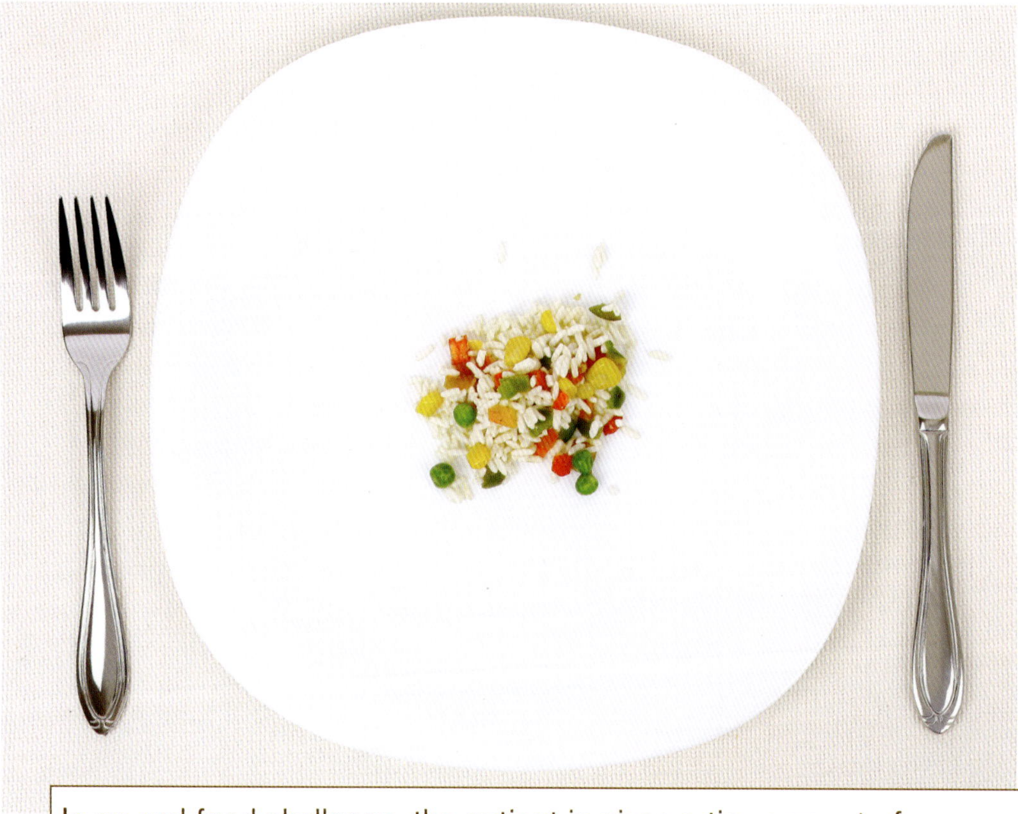

In an oral food challenge, the patient is given a tiny amount of food—much less than someone would normally eat. To prevent bias, the food is sometimes disguised or hidden in another food product.

Knowledge Is Power

Some people get angry, scared, or sad when they are diagnosed with an allergy, and it is not hard to see why. Favorite foods may not only suddenly be off-limits to them—they may even turn out to be deadly. Families that enjoyed going out to eat together may stop doing so for fear that restaurant staff may not take enough care to keep allergens out of

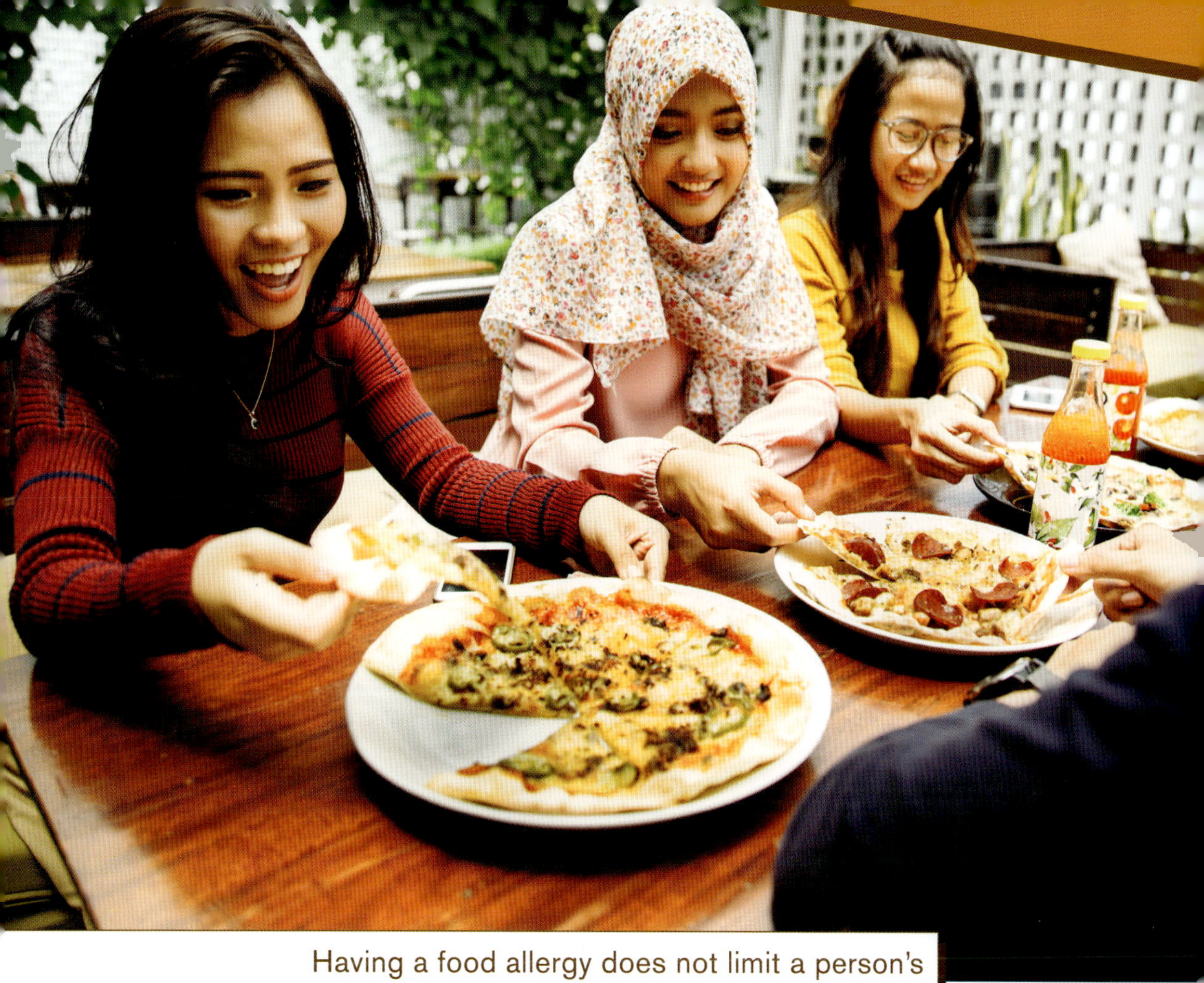

Having a food allergy does not limit a person's potential for happiness.

the meal of the person who was diagnosed. In other cases, however, the results of an allergy test can come as a relief. This is especially true for people who have already had one bad experience with a particular food and are scared to try it again, or who know they are allergic to something but have trouble identifying which ingredient in their food it is. Once they have a diagnosis, their health problems are no longer a mystery to them. Instead, they can make plans and develop strategies that allow them to keep their food allergies at bay as they go about their daily lives.

Chapter Four

LAWS, SCIENCE, AND FOOD PRODUCTION

As the prevalence of food allergies has increased, research and medical organizations have partnered with government agencies to develop programs and laws to address the growing concerns of affected citizens and their loved ones. While researchers attempt to better understand allergies and develop better treatments, support groups may work to spread the latest knowledge while building a community. Still other groups reach out to politicians who can pass laws that better protect those with food allergies.

The Legal System and Food Allergies

Laws that govern things such as food labeling help protect people with allergies from eating foods that are dangerous to them. Other types of laws prevent people with allergies from being discriminated against; for instance, a restaurant cannot refuse to serve someone with allergies. The Rehabilitation Act of 1973 was one of the first laws to partially address food allergies. The law was passed to protect those with mental or physical disabilities from discrimination in both the workplace and schools. Section 504 of the act stated that school children with disabilities had to be included in regular school activities whenever possible.

Although an allergy is not medically classified as a disability, the law included some protections for children with allergies as well. "A 504 plan works well for children with food allergies because it can address lunchroom and classroom policies, general food and hand-washing policies, field trip protocol, and emergency procedures if there is an allergic reaction," explained attorney Tess O'Brien-Heinzen. "Unfortunately, many schools do not regularly evaluate food allergy sufferers under the rubric of the Rehabilitation Act but rather attempt to deal with food allergies on a more informal case-by-case basis."[29]

The next major federal law that had an impact on people with food allergies was the Americans with Disabilities Act (ADA). Passed in 1990, the ADA was the nation's first comprehensive civil rights law for people with disabilities. It required employers, businesses, schools, and government agencies to make sure that they operated in a way that did not discriminate against people with disabilities. Many establishments for children that provide food as part of their services—such as schools, day care centers, and summer camps—made changes to their operations so they could better meet the needs of children with food allergies under the ADA.

As it turned out, though, the U.S. court system did not necessarily believe that either Section 504 or the ADA applied to people with food allergies. To be protected under the ADA, for example, "an individual must prove that he or she is disabled," wrote O'Brien-Heinzen. "This has not been an easy task. Courts have tended to interpret the term narrowly; indeed, individuals with such serious illnesses as AIDS, cancer, and diabetes have been among those found not to have disabilities under the ADA and therefore to not be covered by its protections."[30]

In 1999, the U.S. Eighth Circuit Court decided in the case *Land v. Baptist Medical Center* that a day care center did not have to make special accommodations for a food-allergic preschooler. The Court ruled that even though the preschooler was severely allergic to peanut products, she did not qualify for ADA protection because she could eat other foods safely and could breathe normally except when she was around peanuts and peanut-related foods.

This ruling surprised and outraged families dealing with severe food allergies, but it remained the law of the land for the next several years. In 2008, though, the Americans with Disabilities Act Amendments Act (ADAAA) was passed. This legislation greatly expanded the legal meaning of the term "disability." It stated that the definition of disability should be taken broadly rather than narrowly. In other words, instead of looking for technicalities that would exclude someone from disability coverage, accommodations should be provided for people who need them. Legal experts believe that this new language makes it much easier for people with food allergies, as well as people with mental or physical impairments, to qualify as disabled under the law and receive its protections. Schools and other establishments now have a greater legal obligation to make sure that their facilities are safe and inclusive for children and adults who have food allergies.

Labeling and Instruction for Safer Food

The Food Allergen Labeling and Consumer Protection Act (FALCPA) was enacted in 2006. The act requires easy-to-read warning labels on all packaged food containing protein from any of the eight most common allergen categories. The law immediately lightened the burden for millions of Americans suffering from an allergy to eggs, peanuts, tree nuts, milk, wheat, fish, shellfish, or soybeans.

In January 2011, President Barack Obama signed the Food Allergy & Anaphylaxis Management Act (FAAMA) into law. The law, which was passed as part of a broad set of new national food safety laws and food production regulations, was written in large part by members of FAAN. Its passage marked the end of a long struggle for food allergy advocates. Although FAAMA had first been introduced in Congress in 2005 and had support from both Democrats and Republicans, it never managed to be enacted until 2011.

FAAMA is designed to provide schools across the country with the resources they need to protect students with food allergies. It authorized the federal government to create voluntary national guidance materials for managing food allergies in the country's schools. One of the bill's leading champions was Senator Christopher Dodd, a Democrat from Connecticut whose daughter has been diagnosed with severe food allergies. "All of our nation's children deserve a

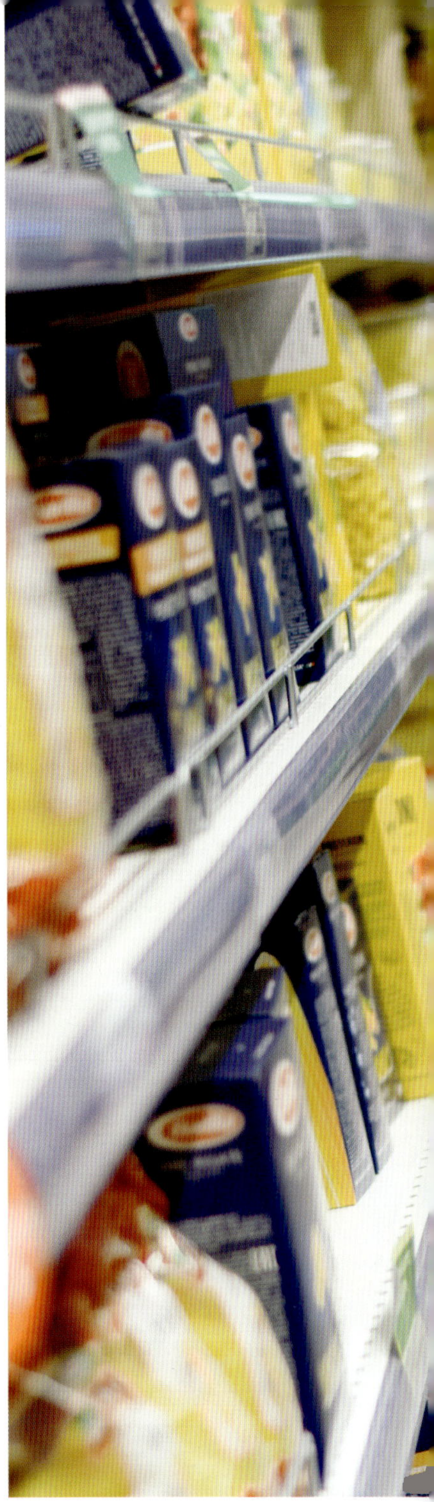

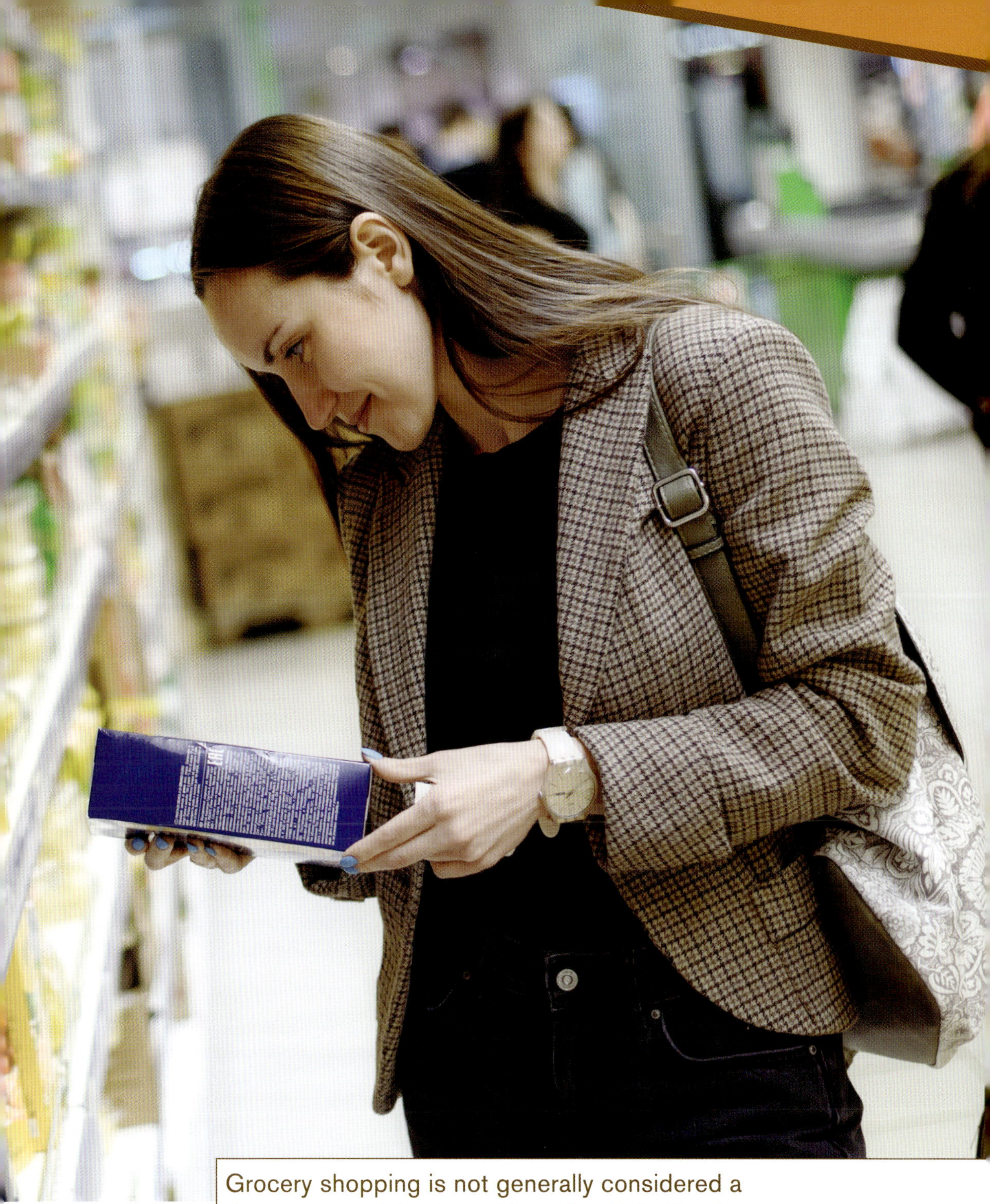

Grocery shopping is not generally considered a dangerous activity, but without food labeling, it would be risky for people with allergies.

No Peanuts at School?

With the number of cases of anaphylactic shock from peanut allergies steadily rising, many schools have decided to limit or ban peanuts and peanut products. In some cases, administrators have established peanut-free rooms or cafeteria tables. In others, they have approved complete bans on having anything with peanuts in it anywhere on school grounds.

These measures have prompted complaints from some parents, who say that outlawing peanut butter and jelly sandwiches makes it harder for them to pack nutritious lunches that their children will eat. The majority of parents and students, though, seem to understand that these bans are necessary. As one parent said, "All kids have a right to be safe in school, and that's something all kids should care about. If by giving up a food you like, you could keep a classmate from getting sick, why wouldn't you want to?"[1]

In addition to instituting peanut butter bans, a few school districts have begun to train teachers, bus drivers, cafeteria workers, and other school employees about how to use epinephrine auto-injectors in case someone does have an allergic reaction. Not everyone can afford an epinephrine auto-injector, but in 2013, President Barack Obama passed a law that gives states financial incentives to pass laws that allow schools to stock epinephrine and make it accessible to all students with allergies, even those who do not have a prescription.

School districts have also made special efforts to educate kids about the risks of severe food allergies. The state of Connecticut, for example, requires teachers to educate their classes about allergies. Supporters believe that these measures not only keep kids with food allergies safer, but also help increase their classmates' support and understanding.

1. "Peanut Butter Jam: Will Food Allergies Kick Your Favorite Snack out of School?," *Weekly Reader (WR), Senior Edition*, October 10, 2008, p. 4.

safe and healthy learning environment," said Dodd. "As a parent of a child who suffers from severe food allergies, I know firsthand the distress this can cause young children and their families. As the number of children with food allergies continues to rise, FAAMA will establish guidelines for the management of food allergies in schools—protecting the well-being of millions of children with life-threatening allergies."[31]

In addition to these federal laws, some states have passed regulations to protect their citizens from exposure to food allergies. In February 2010, for example, Massachusetts passed a law requiring restaurants to educate their staffs about food allergies and to post information and instructions about food allergies in a staff area.

A Closer Look

The School Nutrition Association does not advocate food bans in schools. Instead, it encourages those with food allergies to learn how to manage their allergy.

Searching for a Cure

While medications have been developed to treat allergic reactions, scientists still have not found a cure for food allergies. All over the world, researchers are working to invent new treatments to lessen the burden of living with a food allergy. Geneticists hope that one day they could develop therapies to stop individuals from ever developing an allergy in the first place.

One of the most promising of these areas of study is called immunotherapy. This process involves changing the behavior of the immune system so that it no longer attacks harmless particles. Immunotherapy is already being used with a fair amount of success for treating other types of allergies. For instance, immunotherapy for pollen allergies involves injecting small amounts of highly diluted pollen under the skin so the body gets used to it and does not see higher amounts as a threat.

For food allergies, instead of injections, the immunotherapy process involves giving allergic people extremely tiny amounts of the food to which they are allergic. The researchers then very gradually increase the dose of the food the patients receive. This process, known as oral immunotherapy, takes place under extremely close medical supervision in case of any severe allergic reaction. In some of these tests, people with food allergies have shown an increased ability to consume foods that have always given them severe problems in the past. Another type of treatment, called sublingual immunotherapy, involves giving patients the allergen in liquid form under the tongue. As with oral

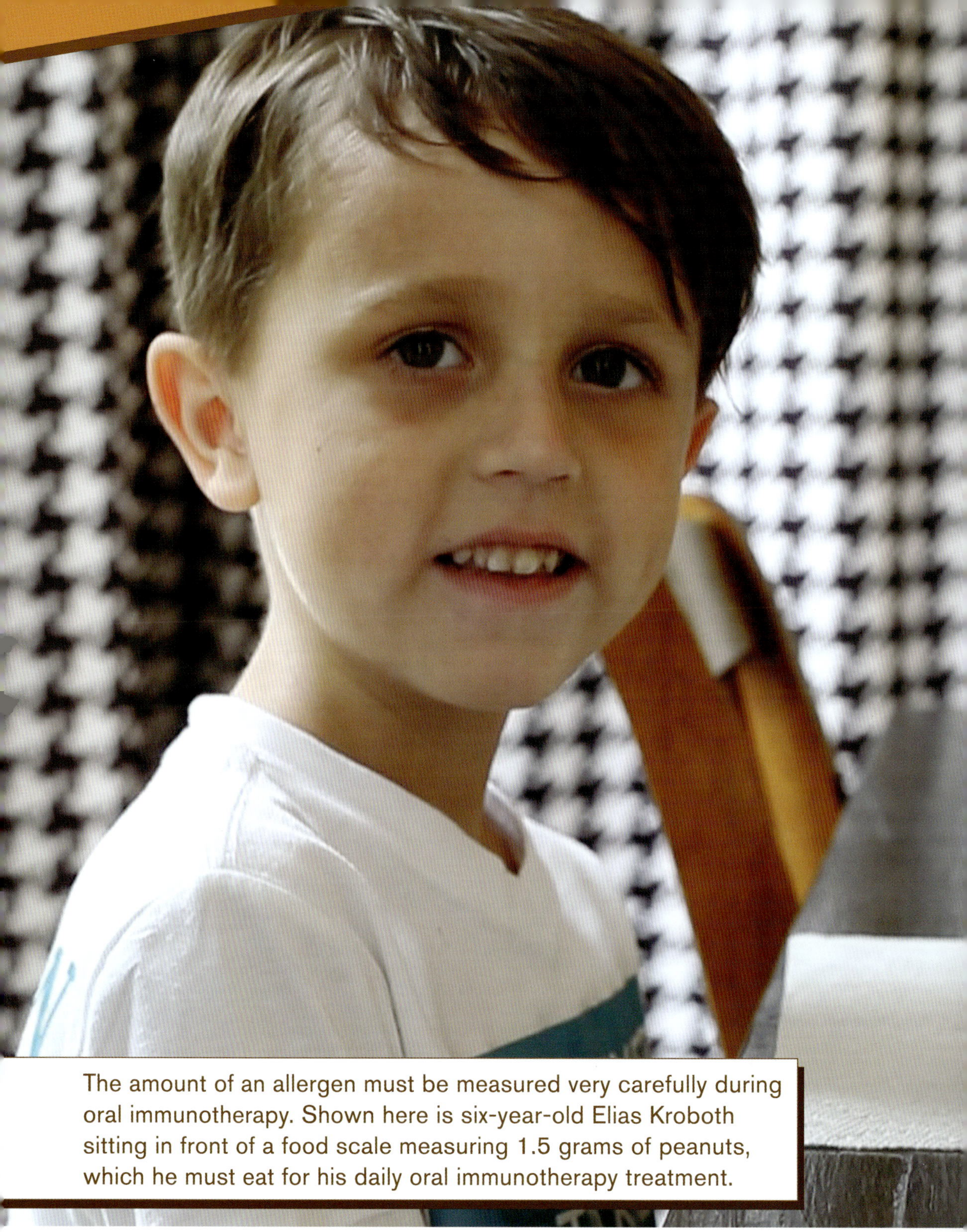

The amount of an allergen must be measured very carefully during oral immunotherapy. Shown here is six-year-old Elias Kroboth sitting in front of a food scale measuring 1.5 grams of peanuts, which he must eat for his daily oral immunotherapy treatment.

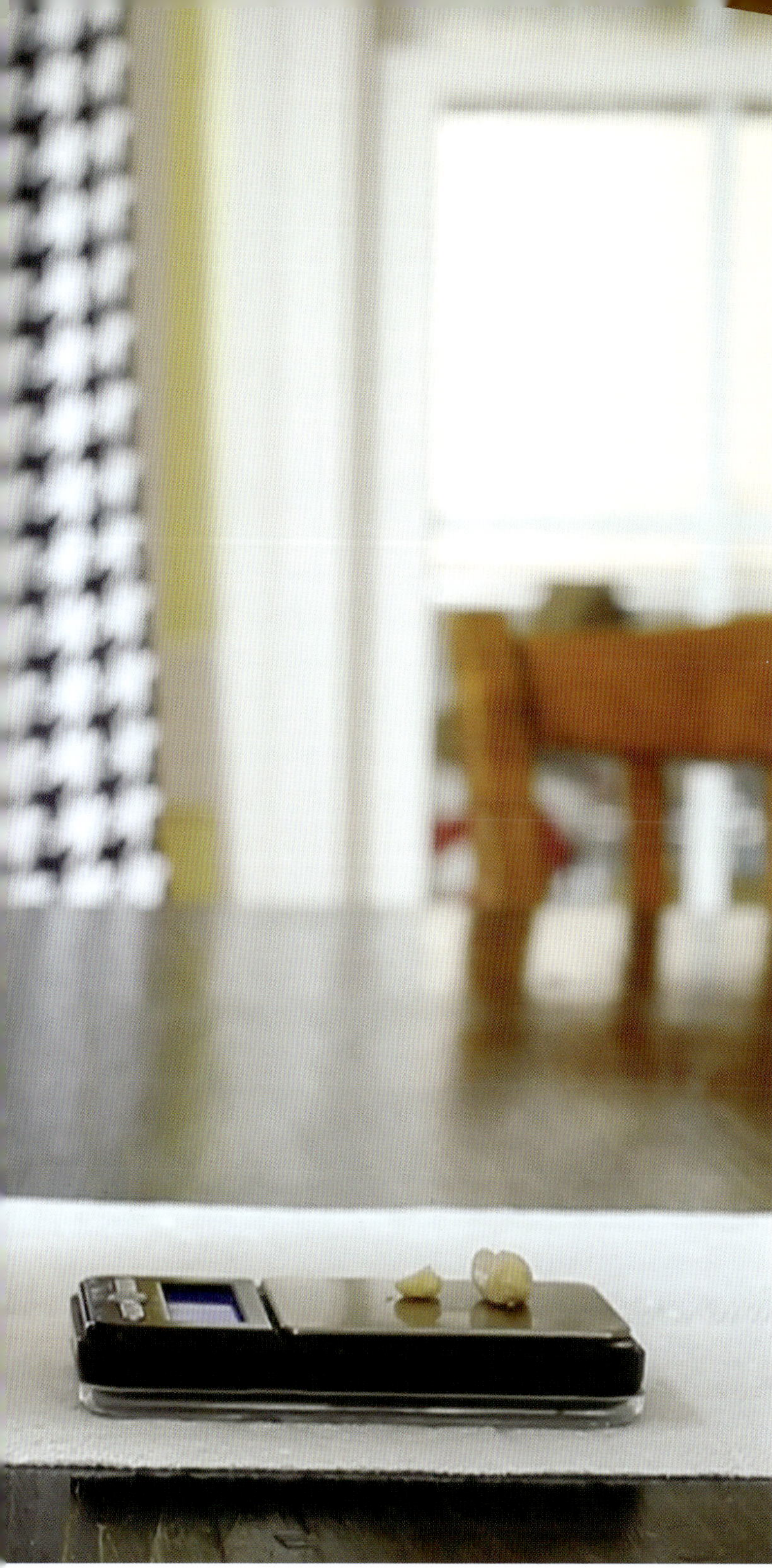

immunotherapy, the doses are gradually increased. Patients have reported fewer side effects with sublingual immunotherapy when compared with oral immunotherapy.

Although some people have had positive results with both types of immunotherapy, more research is needed before it can become a widespread treatment. According to the AAAAI, many questions remain: "How long does desensitization last? Do patients eventually achieve complete tolerance of the allergen? Do patients [stick to] their regular dosing of the allergen? What happens if they stop eating the allergen?"[32] There are indications, for example, that immunotherapy may only work if participants receive their oral or sublingual dose on a daily or almost daily basis. Otherwise, the allergic reactions intensify again, and all the earlier progress that the patient made is lost. However, the only long-term studies that have been done as of 2019 have been small, so their results cannot necessarily be trusted to apply to the general population.

Nonetheless, many allergists are extremely excited about the treatment advances they have already made. According to Laura Beil,

> *If nothing else, the experiments have shown for the first time that curing food allergies is at least possible … Some children who began studies with immune reactions to even the smallest trace of peanut can now eat up to 13 nuts in one sitting. Similar dramatic gains have been seen for milk and egg allergies. Only a few children have been involved in each study so far, but researchers are cautiously increasing the number of enrollees.*[33]

Allergists are investigating other approaches as well in their quest to free people from food allergies. For example, scientists are experimenting with genetic food allergy vaccines, also sometimes called DNA immunizations. Under this program, a scientist might create a vaccine for peanut allergies, for example, by injecting genes with coding for peanut protein directly into immune system cells. Such a genetic change would get the immune system cells to make the protein themselves, eliminating the body's immune response when the protein comes into the body through food. "The idea behind DNA immunization is that when the body produces the allergen from within,

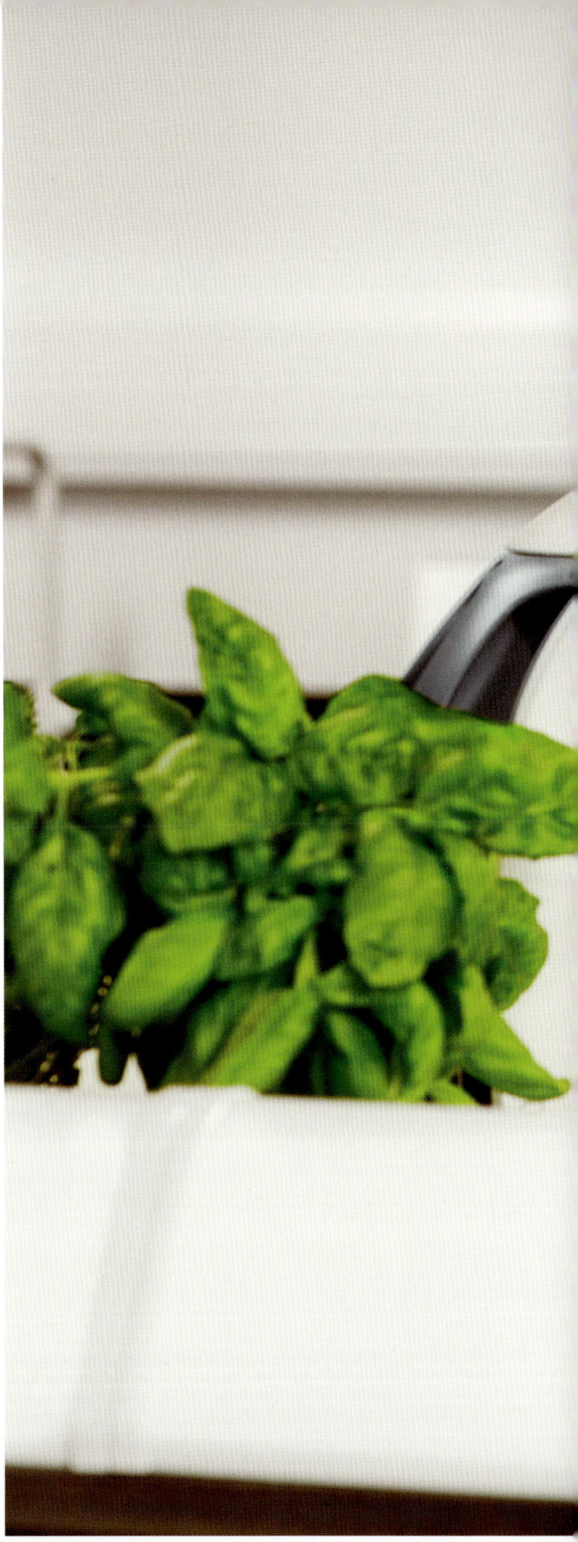

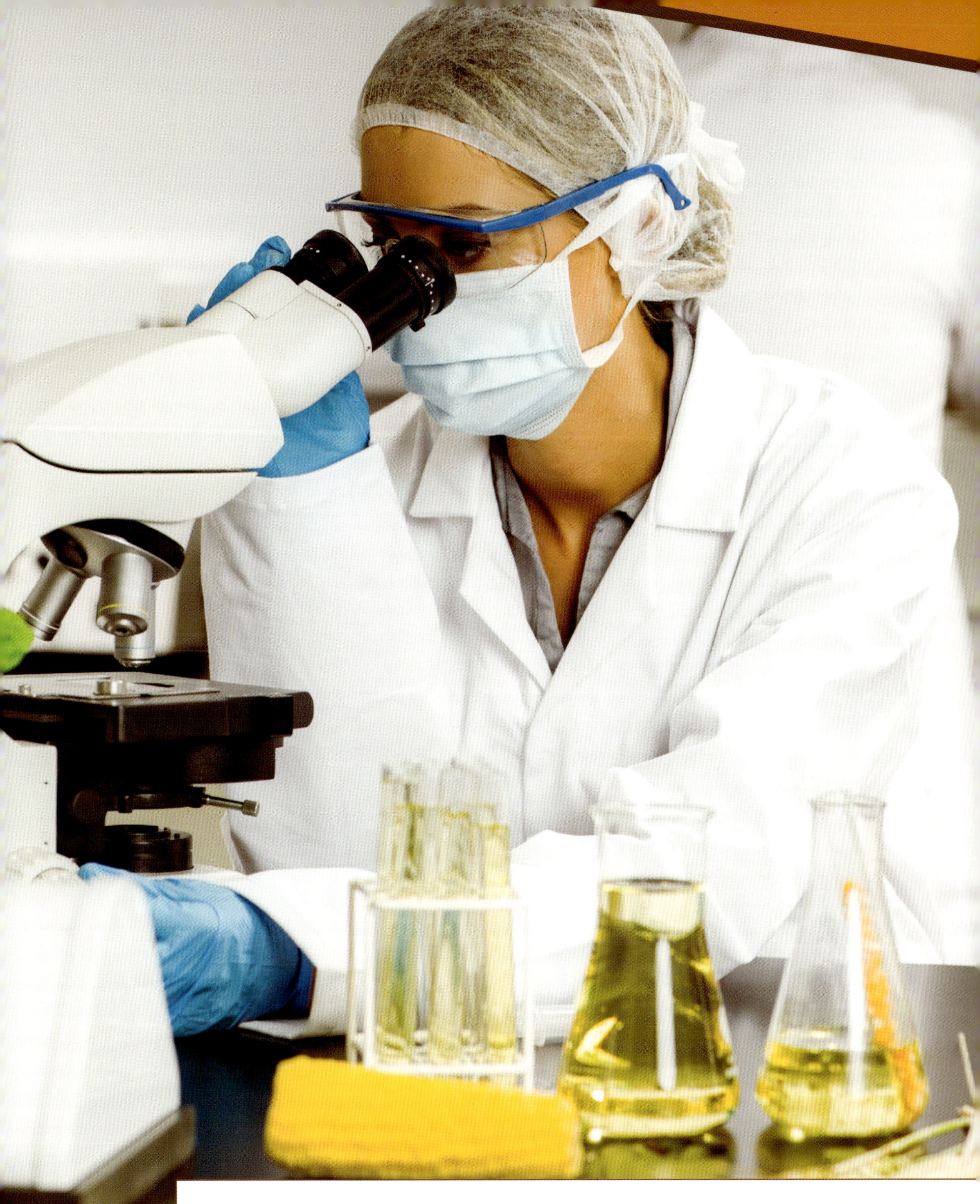

Scientists continue to research new ways to treat food allergies.

the immune system no longer views the allergen as a foreign invader, and hence has no reason to attack it," explained Robert A. Wood. "This therapy is far from ready for human experimentation, but similar strategies are being used to treat other diseases in people, including cystic fibrosis and sickle cell disease, so this may not be as far fetched as it sounds."[34]

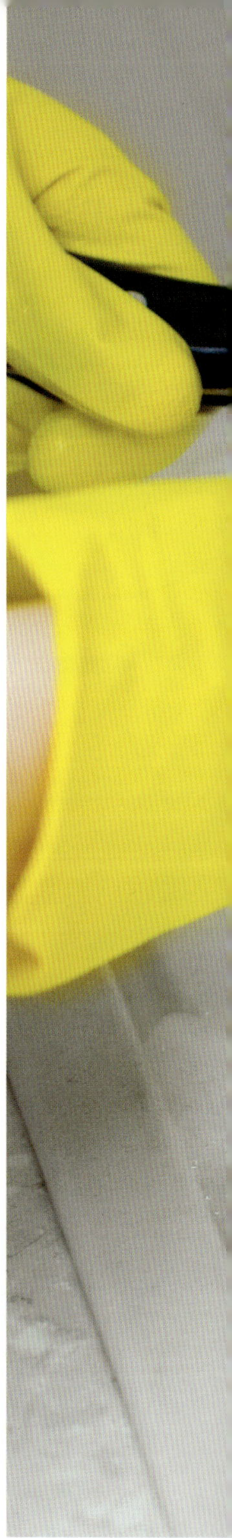

A Closer Look

According to a 2016 study by Rush University, race does not play a large role in allergies; peanuts were the number one food allergen among black, Latinx, and white children.

Even the most optimistic researchers admit, though, that finding a permanent cure for food allergies will require years of additional study and experimentation. The challenge, according to Claudia Kalb, is that "while scientists have a basic understanding of how allergies work, they can still be stumped by the immune system, which is too complex to submit easily to their control."[35] Until more progress is made in this area, the best people with food allergies can do is avoid their allergens, which is why it is important for people with and without allergies to learn as much as they can about them.

Cross Contamination and Government Regulation

Cross contamination is a potentially dangerous occurrence that can happen anywhere food is processed or prepared. Cross contamination is when a food item that is not an allergen comes in direct contact with a food item that is an allergen. The problems that can arise from cross contamination make it a major concern for the entire food industry. Farmers, factory workers, delivery drivers, grocery store employees, and restaurant workers must all work to avoid cross contamination. Because of this, new technology and better processing protocols for safe food handling are in constant development. Cross contamination most frequently occurs at home or in

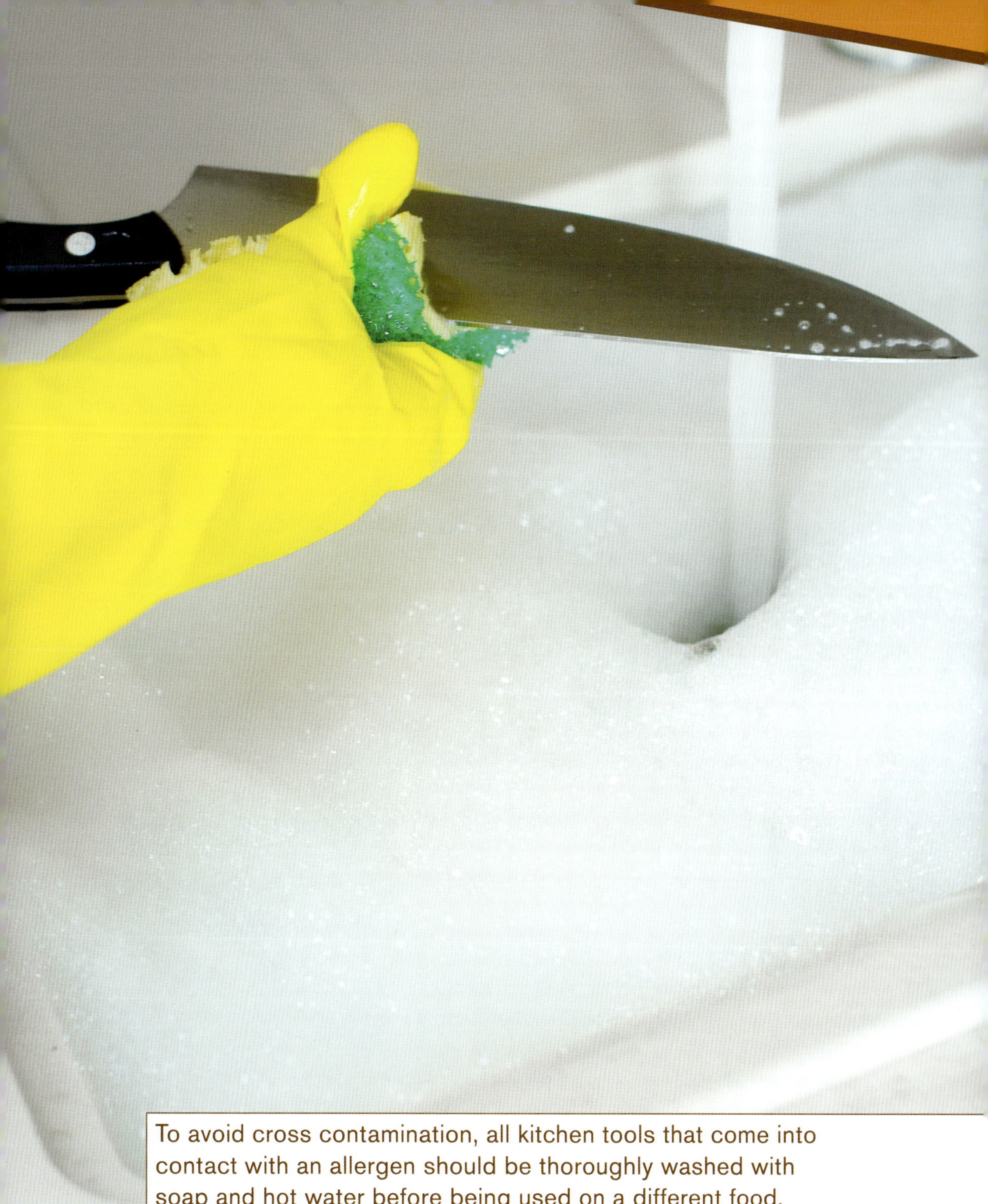

To avoid cross contamination, all kitchen tools that come into contact with an allergen should be thoroughly washed with soap and hot water before being used on a different food. If possible, a completely different utensil should be used.

restaurant kitchens. It generally happens when a knife, cutting board, bowl, or other kitchen implement is used to prepare an allergenic food, then comes into contact with a previously "safe" food before being washed or otherwise sanitized. The safe food thus becomes tainted with residue from the allergenic food to the point that it, too, can trigger health problems when it is eaten.

Food-processing companies face this same challenge, except on a much bigger scale. Many food-production facilities manufacture a variety of different food items that appear on supermarket shelves. If they are not careful in their operations, huge volumes of food can become contaminated with allergens in a matter of minutes. This is why, for the safety of people with allergies, the package of a nonallergenic food may have a label on it noting that it was processed in a factory that also processes allergenic foods. Fortunately for food makers and their customers, many food industries have developed advanced systems to shield their operations from accidental contamination from food allergens. The ice cream industry is a good example. According to a 2006 article in *Food Engineering* magazine,

> *Ice cream manufacturers typically produce both nonallergenic and allergenic products on the same [production] lines. They are dipping into technology's equipment arsenal to cope with the allergen-control challenge. Dreyer's Grand Ice Cream installed more than 100 mix-proof valves at its Bakersfield, CA, plant to enhance its ability to clean out egg, peanut, and other allergen residues from lines before a nonallergenic product is run.*[36]

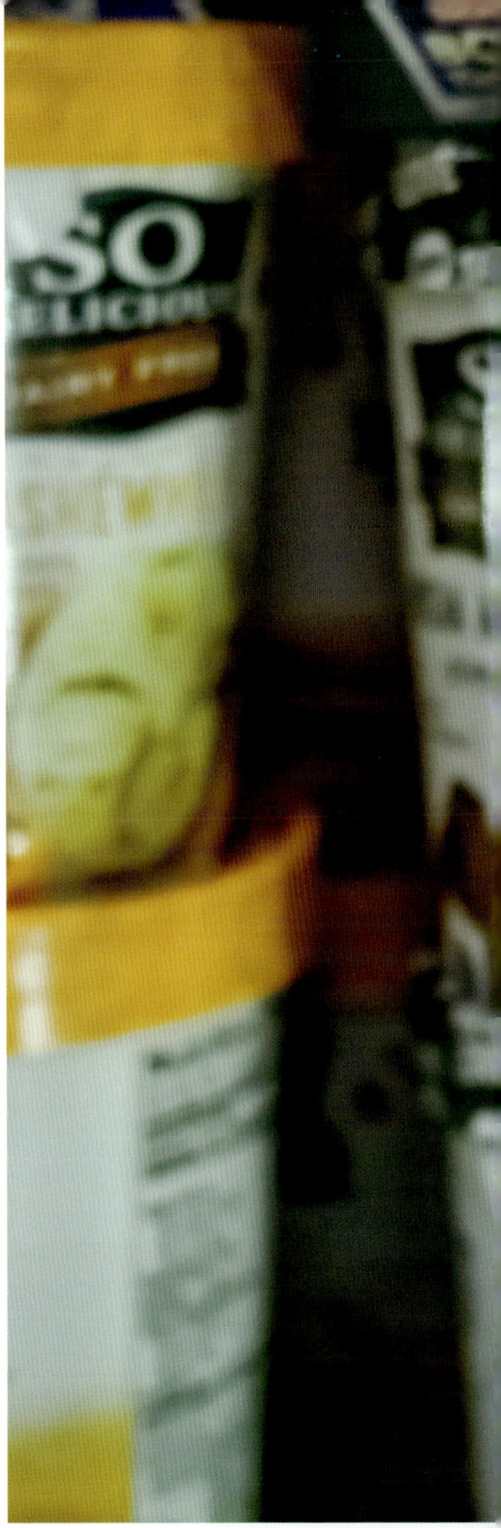

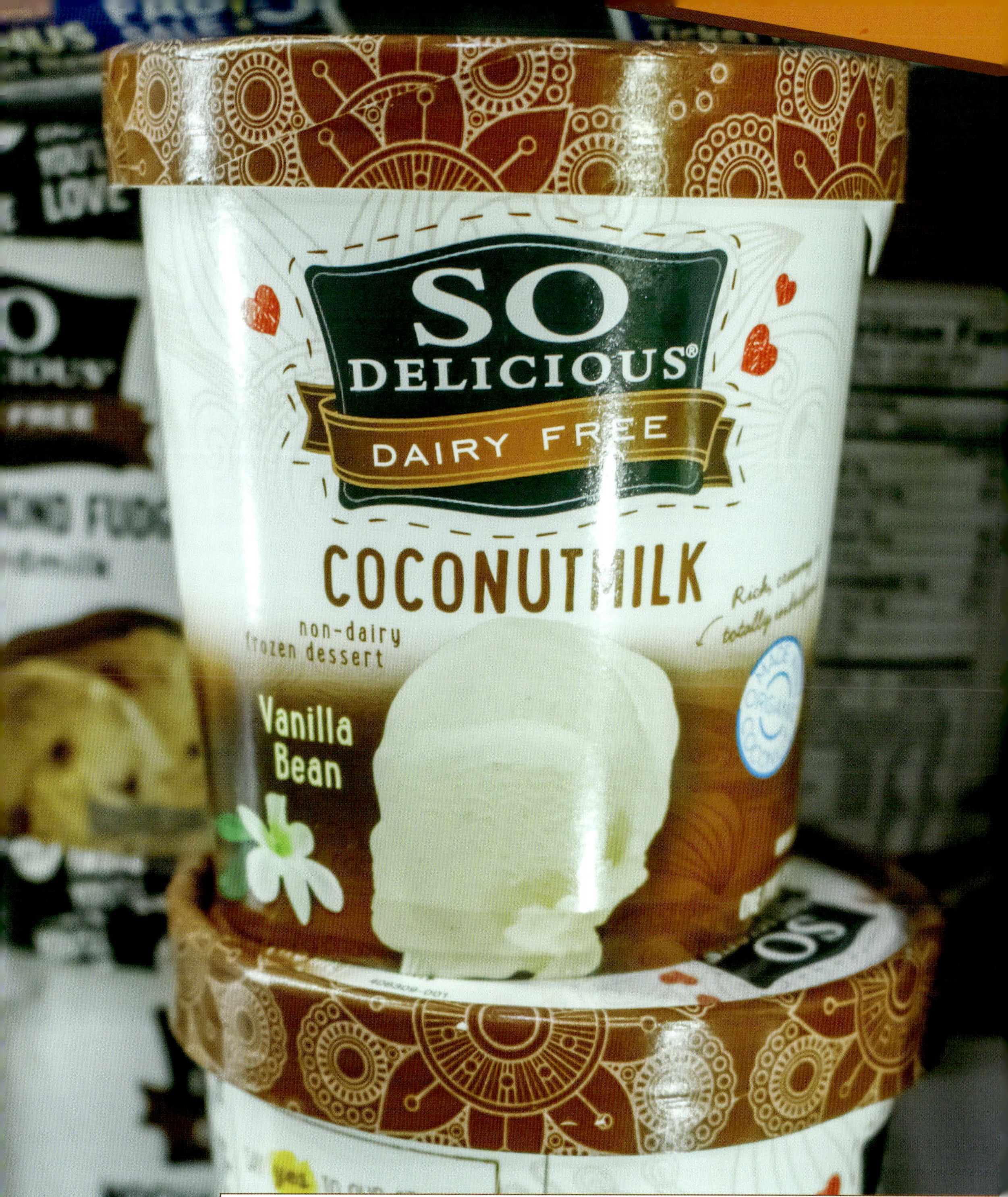

Foods that are free of a common allergen are generally clearly labeled.

Companies that avoid cross contamination and properly label their food products can obtain significant business benefits in the long run. "It all boils down to trust," said Anne Muñoz-Furlong. "If people affected by food allergies trust the information they are given, they will trust that product, and they become very brand loyal and tell everyone else."[37]

Chapter Five

LIVING LIFE TO ITS FULLEST

Once someone is diagnosed with a severe food allergy, new commitments are required from every member of the family. Day-to-day living must change, but not necessarily for the worse. While challenges will present themselves at every meal and outing, a little planning will go a long way. For those prone to anaphylactic reactions, using common sense and always having an epinephrine injector handy will quickly become a way of life.

In addition to the physical effects they have, food allergies have the potential to take a heavy toll on one's social life. Food allergies can lead to arguments between teens seeking independence and parents who are fearful of the many different ways that their child might be accidentally exposed to allergens. Food allergies can also put up walls between kids and their peers. Some classmates might resent rules that do not allow them to bring some of their favorite foods to school. Others may not understand food allergies, so they might avoid kids who have them as if the condition were contagious.

Finally, food allergies can become a weapon in the hands of bullies. A woman named Jyoti told the website The Mighty about an incident that happened to her seven-year-old daughter, Jaya. Jyoti wrote that "a classmate was waving a cheese string to which she is allergic around her. She asked him to stop and he refused … After school Jaya said she wants to go to an 'allergy school' to be with other kids like her who understand what it's like to live with food allergies."[38] While some adults say children should stand up to or avoid bullies who hurt their feelings, someone with an allergy does not have the option to "just ignore" someone who is waving their allergen in their face.

What Not to Say

Sometimes people say or do things that are hurtful or frustrating to people with allergies simply because they are not fully informed about them. For example, someone who knows a person with a sensitivity to strawberries that they call an allergy may say to someone with a true allergy, "My other friend is allergic to strawberries, but she still eats them." Someone may also put an allergen near the person who is allergic; sometimes this is a way to bully others and purposely upset them, but other times it is an attempt at a joke, and the person may not understand why their allergic friend is so angry about it. Other things people should avoid saying to someone with an allergy include:

- "Will you die if you eat this food?"
- "A little bit of [allergen] won't hurt you."
- "Just take some over-the-counter allergy medicine and you'll be fine."
- "If you eat your allergen, it'll cure your allergy."
- "It's not my fault you're allergic; why shouldn't I be able to eat what I want around you?"
- "It's all in your head. You could eat it if you wanted to."
- "Are you just saying that because you don't like [allergen]/are just trying to lose weight/have an eating disorder?"
- "Have you tried [yoga/essential oils/cutting out other foods]?"
- "You just want attention."
- "If you don't eat this, you'll hurt my feelings."
- "I would hate my life if I couldn't eat [allergen]."
- "Why do you have to be so difficult?"
- "You have your auto-injector, so just use it after you eat [allergen]."
- "There's [allergen] in that food you're eating … Just kidding!"

A bully who uses a food allergy against someone is doing something very harmful and dangerous.

Despite all these additional challenges, though, tens of thousands of kids and adults with significant food allergies are able to lead happy and productive lives. Armed with confidence and knowledge,

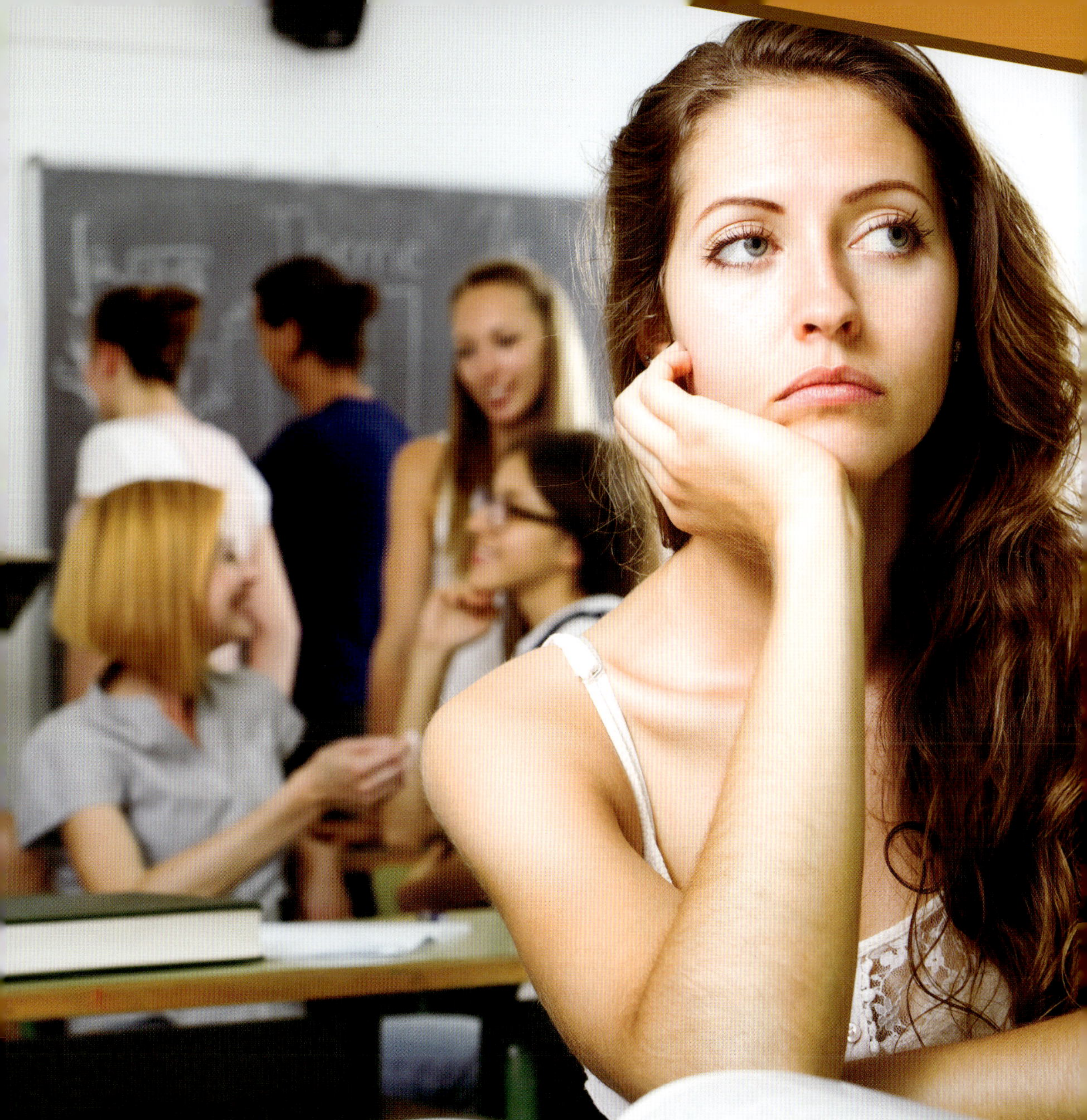

When people do not fully understand allergies, they may unintentionally isolate people who have them. For example, sometimes people with allergies are not invited to parties because other people do not want to worry about feeding them something that will cause an allergic reaction. This can make it harder for someone to make friends with their classmates.

they refuse to allow food allergies to define them or keep them from pursuing their dreams and having fun.

The Importance of Social Acceptance

Young children who have severe food allergies generally do not spend a lot of time worrying about whether their condition will lead to rejection from other kids. As kids get older, though, their awareness of social situations increases. It is here that special food rules for certain kids come to their attention. It is also during this stage of development that many young adults become extremely uncomfortable with the idea of being different from their peers in any way. They want to fit in and not draw attention to themselves. For many young people with severe food allergies, this can make them start to view their allergies as a source of embarrassment and discomfort.

In some cases, the feelings of embarrassment over their condition can lead teens with food allergies to adopt self-destructive attitudes. "I've had patients who've literally said they'd rather die than use an EpiPen," said Calman Prussin, a researcher with the National Institute of Allergy and Infectious Diseases. "And I wonder: Where did they get that message?"[39]

Some kids with severe food allergies say that their own personal attitude toward their medical condition can make a big difference in how other kids perceive them. "The number one fear for many of those who live with food allergies is not the fear of having a reaction, but the fear of being accepted," wrote Annie Jorgensen, winner of the Miss Wisconsin Outstanding Teen scholarship pageant in 2011. She continued,

> *It has been my personal experience that others are more accepting of your food allergy once you have accepted [it] yourself. I believe this is achieved when you are fully prepared and confident in any social situation. Attitude is contagious—if you are comfortable in your own skin, challenges and all, others around you will embrace your food allergies and will be open to learning how to keep you safe.*[40]

Many kids with food allergies also find that their worries about being accepted by classmates and teammates are not based in reality.

Learning How to Self-Advocate

An important part of growing up with a medical issue is learning how to deal with it. This sounds simple, but in fact, it can take time for people to learn the best ways to take care of themselves. For example, a 2006 survey conducted by allergists found that many teens with a history of severe food allergies have a habit of trying food without adequately investigating whether it is safe for them. This may be because they do not want to appear difficult or picky. However, it is important for people with food allergies to get comfortable standing up for themselves, asking to see all the ingredients in a food they have not tried before, and letting others know what allergenic foods cannot be eaten around them. People who take offense to these self-advocacy actions should remember that a person's life can depend on them.

Many teens also admit to leaving their auto-injectors at home because they feel embarrassed about needing them. When combined with risk-taking behavior such as not checking the ingredients in their food, this can have disastrous results. In 2015, *Allergic Living* magazine reported the story of Sydney Harris, a teen who said that when she was first diagnosed with allergies, she "didn't want to be different … I would leave the house without an EpiPen, or put myself in situations where I was at risk. I didn't want to accept that I had food allergies."[1] She stopped doing this when she had to be rushed to the hospital after experiencing anaphylactic shock at a restaurant. Studies have found that support from friends can reduce this type of risky behavior.

1. Quoted in Heather Hewett, "Food Allergy Meets the Teenage Brain," *Allergic Living*, November 23, 2015. www.allergicliving.com/2015/11/23/food-allergy-meets-the-teenage-brain/.

Fourteen-year-old Caitlin, for example, was very excited when she made the junior varsity (JV) volleyball team at her high school. When she realized that she would have to tell not only her JV teammates and coaches but also the varsity squad about her severe allergies to peanuts and tree nuts, though, she became extremely nervous. "I wasn't sure if they would understand [but] I knew that I had to let them know eventually and that it was important for my safety," she recalled.

As it turned out, all the players and coaches were supportive. "All through the season, the team was wonderful in helping me manage my allergy on the bus, at away games, and during special events, such as senior night or team sleepovers. I was lucky to be with such a nice group of people, but also proud of myself for taking charge and keeping myself safe … It opened my eyes to how considerate other teens can be about allergies."[41]

Unfortunately, some young adults learn that people are not as understanding and accepting as Caitlin's teammates and coaches were.

Turn It Teal

Turn It Teal is a food allergy awareness campaign started in 2014 by Stephanie Lowe of Cleveland, Ohio. Every year during Food Allergy Awareness Week in May, buildings, bridges, and other landmarks are lit with teal lights to bring awareness to the issue of food allergies. In 2017, more than 40 landmarks participated.

Teal is the official color of food allergy awareness, and it can be used in other ways as well. For example, anyone can participate in the Teal Pumpkin Project at Halloween. Trick-or-treating is an activity most children enjoy, but for someone with food allergies, it can be disappointing; many types of candy either contain allergens or are processed in a factory that also processes allergenic foods. To allow kids with food allergies to participate in Halloween activities, many people paint a pumpkin teal and leave it outside their house to indicate that they have non-food treats available for children with food allergies. These can include things such as glow sticks, bubbles, kazoos, or bouncy balls. People can also add their house to an interactive map on the FARE website so trick-or-treaters with allergies can find participating houses more easily.

Other holidays are starting to be given the teal treatment too. In February 2019, the Food Allergy & Anaphylaxis Connection Team (FAACT) published a blog post about Valentine's Day, reminding people that students frequently bring in candy for their classmates on this day. FAACT recommended talking to the teacher and asking if students could bring in non-food treats only or be given a list of safe food items. It takes very little effort for people to make sure holidays are fun and inclusive for everyone—even people with food allergies.

The key to handling these difficult experiences is to maintain a sense of self-worth and seek out peers who will accept them for who they are, allergies and all.

Some people are not bothered at all by their allergies. Instead of dwelling on the things they cannot have, they seek out fun activities that do not involve food. However, for others, it is difficult not to feel anxious or depressed. Nicole Smith, a mother of a child with allergies, offered this advice to other families: "If you or your child are experiencing debilitating food allergy anxiety, where depression is setting in

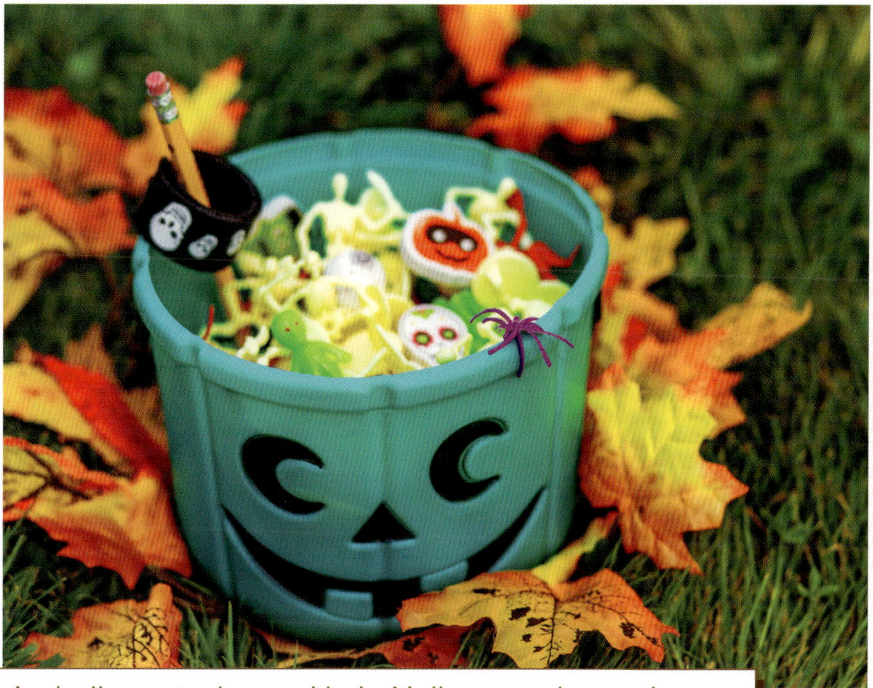

Including a teal pumpkin in Halloween decorations is a simple way to indicate that non-food treats are available for trick-or-treaters. For people who do not have a pumpkin available, printable signs can be downloaded for free from the FARE website and placed on a door or window to alert trick-or-treaters.

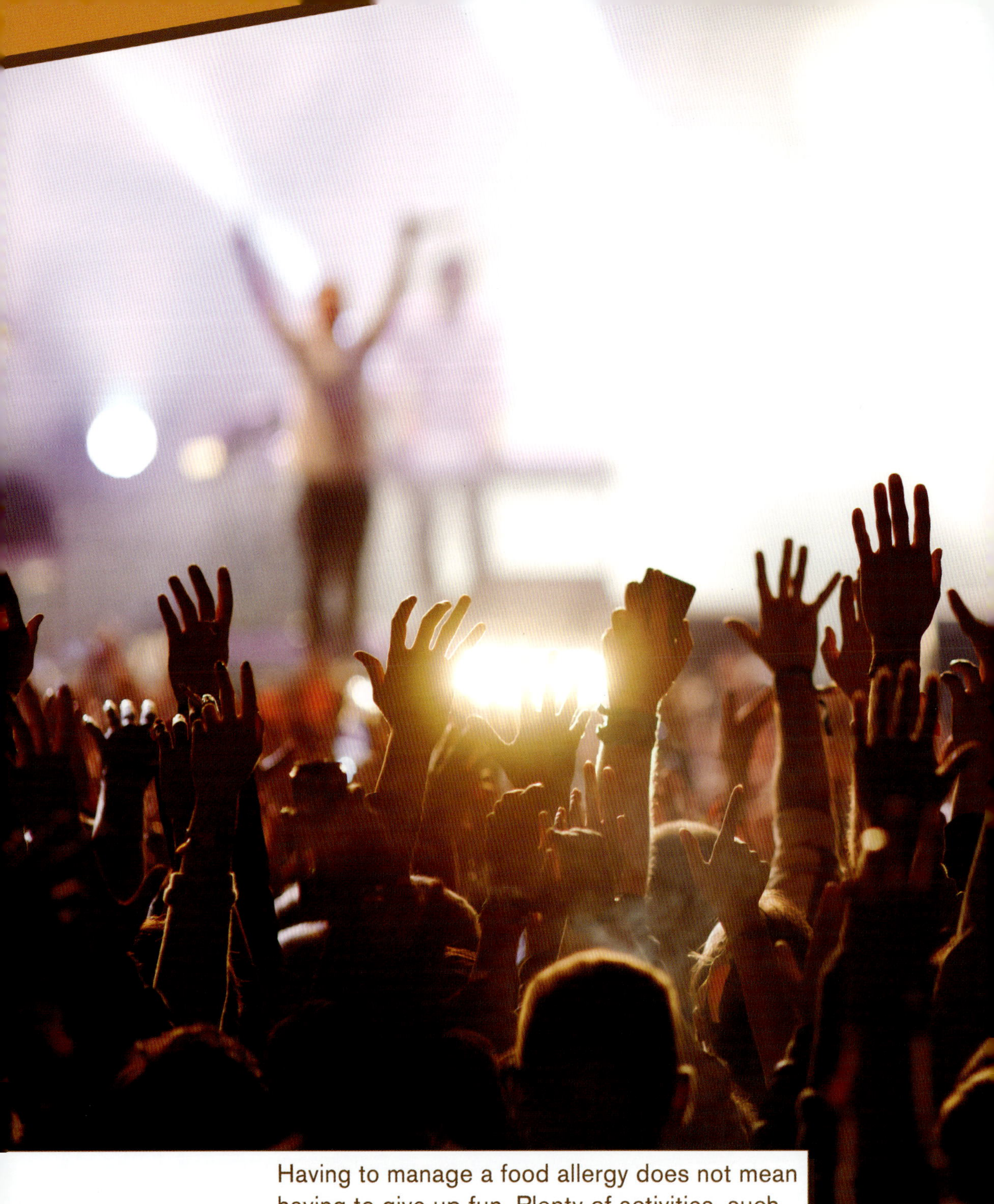

Having to manage a food allergy does not mean having to give up fun. Plenty of activities, such as going to concerts, do not involve food at all.

and/or eating is becoming a difficulty for your child, I'd like to suggest: Share your feelings with a professional! You don't need to suffer, nor does your child. Some of the strongest people I know ask for help."[42]

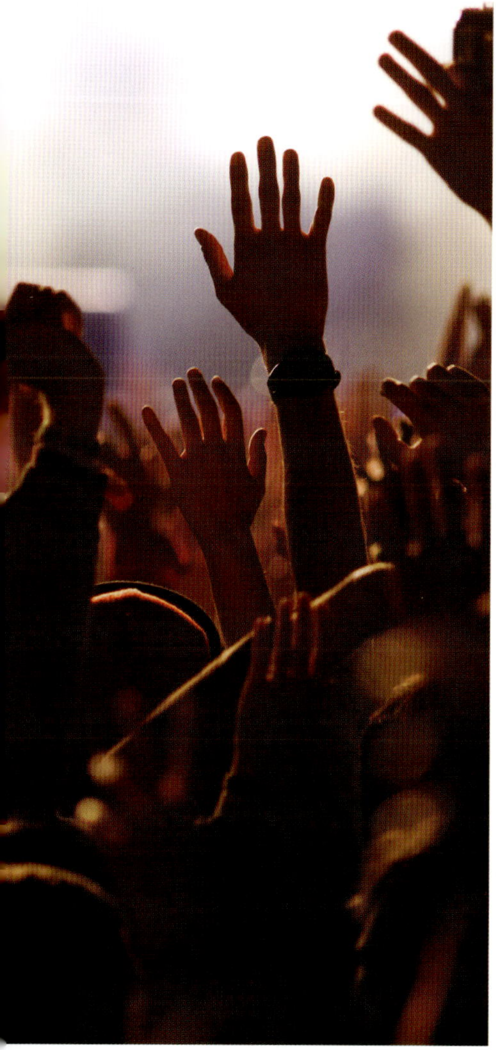

The Joy of Cooking

One of the biggest challenges many people with food allergies face is how to find food that is both tasty and safe to eat outside the home. Whereas people without food allergies can go anywhere and eat anything without worrying about their safety, the stakes for food allergy sufferers are far higher. Some people who have to deal with multiple serious food allergies limit their exposure to foods outside of the home. They either eat most of their meals at home or bring their own prepared food with them wherever they go. Allergists say that for children who are still learning about allergy triggers in foods, these precautions are not only sensible but also necessary.

It is worth noting, however, that dietary options for people with food allergies have expanded greatly in recent years. Entire cookbooks and websites are now devoted to making allergen-free meals and snacks. In addition, food manufacturers have noticed the rising number of people with food allergies over the last decade or so, and they have rushed to attract these consumers with a variety of new products. "Companies have created lots of good substitutes for favorite foods," confirmed KidsHealth. "Everything from dairy-free mashed potatoes to wheat-free chocolate chunk cookies!"[43]

These expanded supermarket offerings have made life much easier for families dealing with

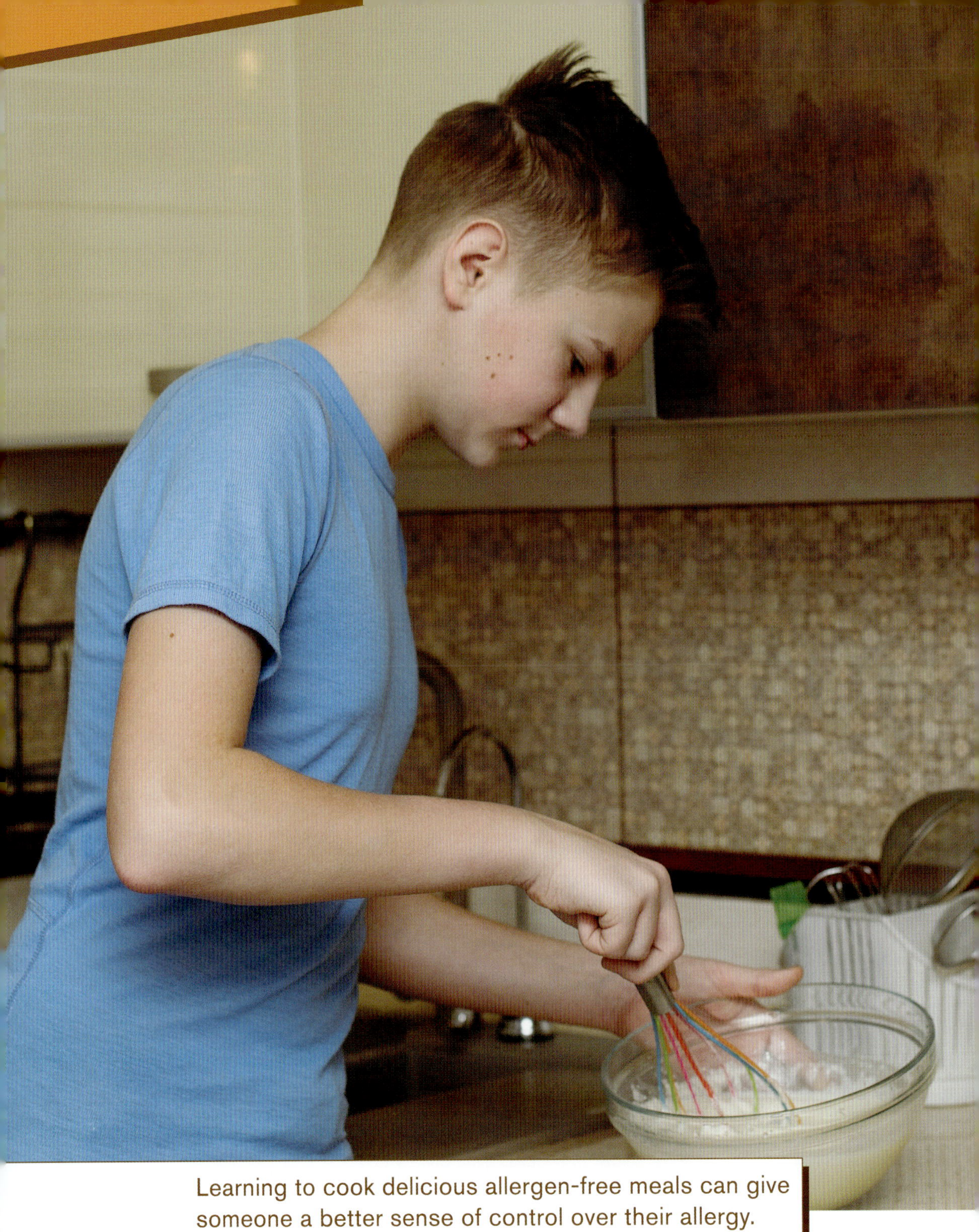

Learning to cook delicious allergen-free meals can give someone a better sense of control over their allergy.

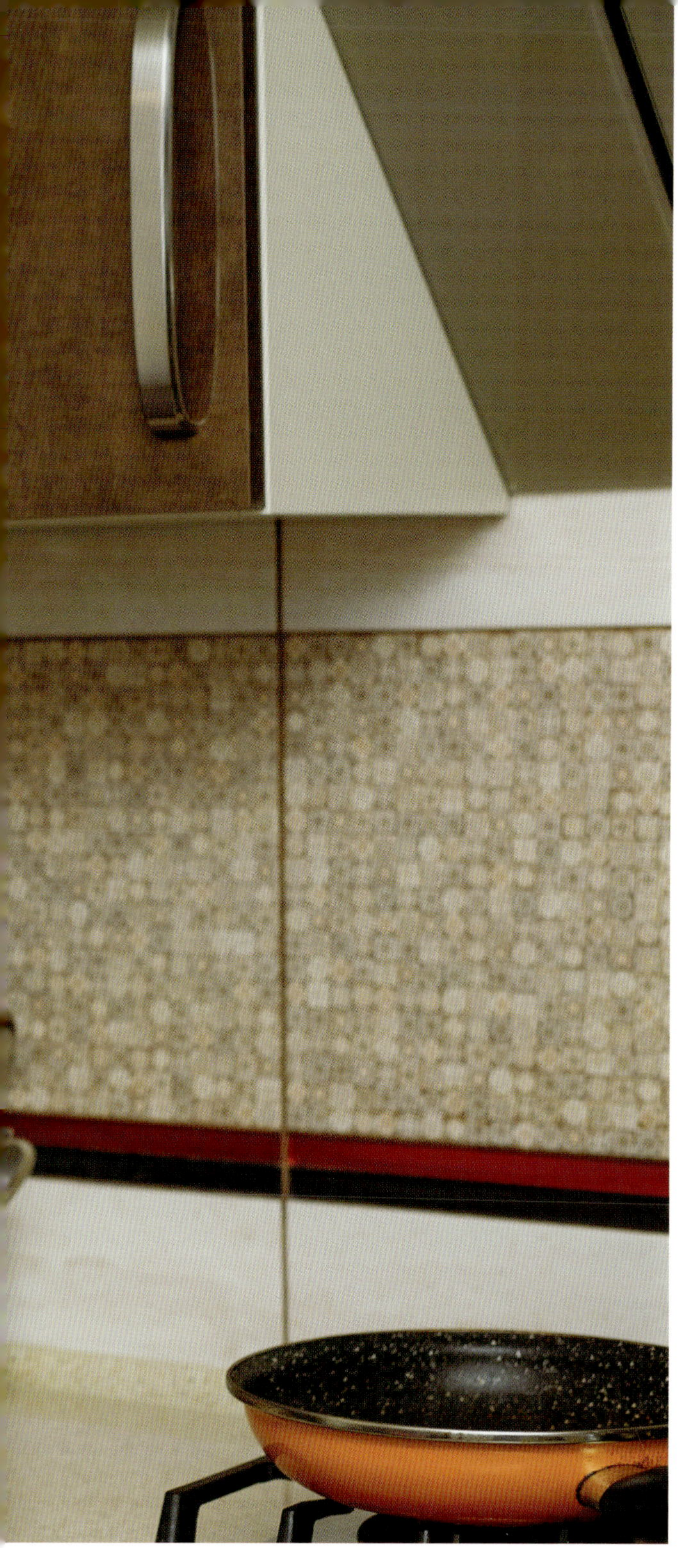

food allergies. However, parents with kids who have allergies still have to read food labels very closely to look for problem ingredients, and they admit that dealing with food allergies is a big hassle. Some of them say, though, that food shopping and meal making gets a lot easier over time.

Pete Wells recalled that when his son Dexter was diagnosed with multiple food allergies, it seemed like there were hardly any foods left that the family could make for him. "He was a year old when we learned he would have to avoid tuna, clams, and shrimp," said Wells. "And onions. And garlic. Peanuts, almonds, walnuts and cashews. Sesame and poppy seeds. Egg whites, chickpeas, and lentils. Soybeans and anything containing soy, which by itself put about half the supermarket off limits."[44] As the months passed, though, Wells and his wife learned more about food allergies, expanded their cooking horizons, and became skilled at substituting ingredients. By the time Dexter was in preschool, they were making eggless cupcakes, pancakes, and meatballs that were just as tasty as the traditional versions—and, according to Wells, it was much easier to do than he had expected.

Going Out to Eat

For middle school and high school students, eating every meal at home is often not a realistic option. Between classes, after-school jobs, extracurricular activities, dating, and other social events, young adults with food allergies spend long periods of time out of the house.

Although people with allergies can—and often do—carry safe snacks with them, most of them also enjoy eating out at restaurants and friends' houses. In addition to getting to eat different foods than they typically make at home, eating with others is a fun, social experience; many people feel uncomfortable being the only person at a table not eating, and most restaurants do not allow people to bring in their own food. Allergists say that as long as people take steps to ensure that the food they are eating is safe for them, there is nothing wrong with eating out. For example, people with food allergies should notify wait staff of their condition, and they should not be afraid to personally speak with kitchen staff to let them know about special food requirements. According to 18-year-old Julie, who is allergic to milk and other dairy products,

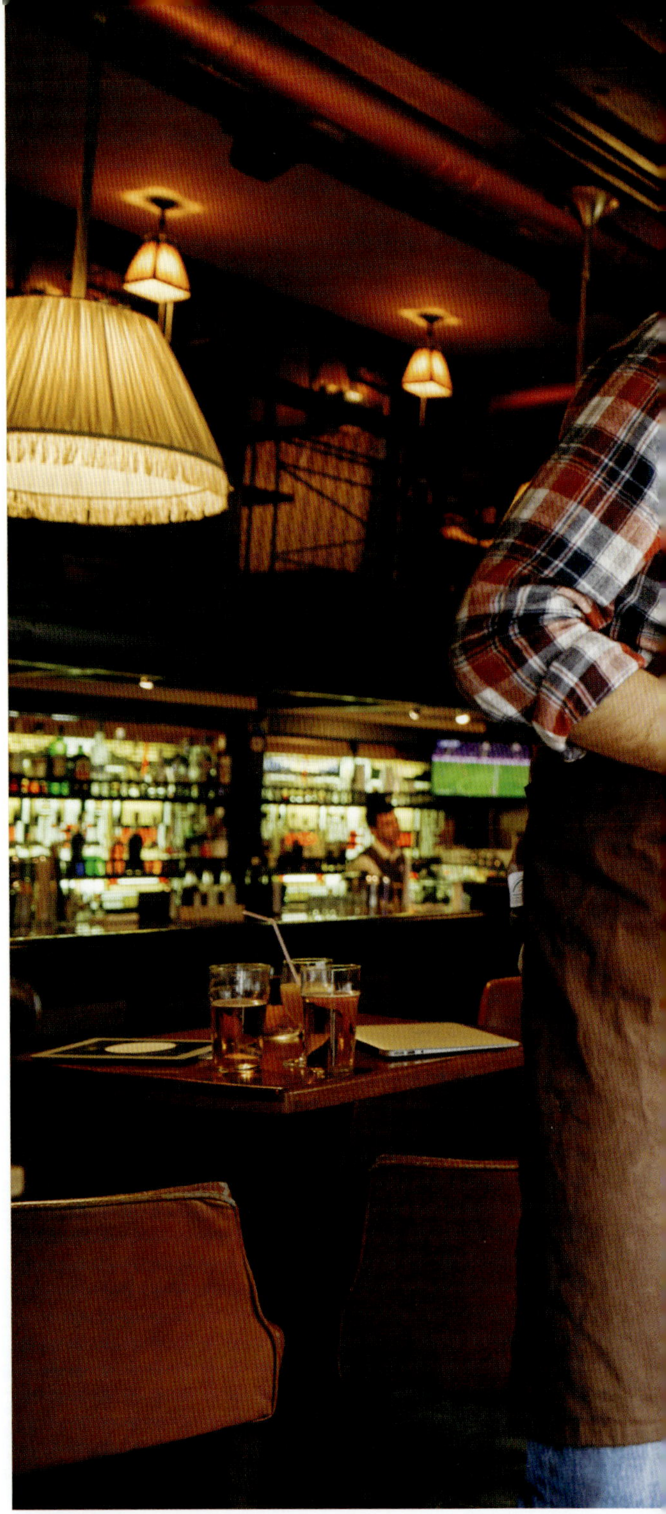

> *Eating out with a food allergy can be a challenge. However,*

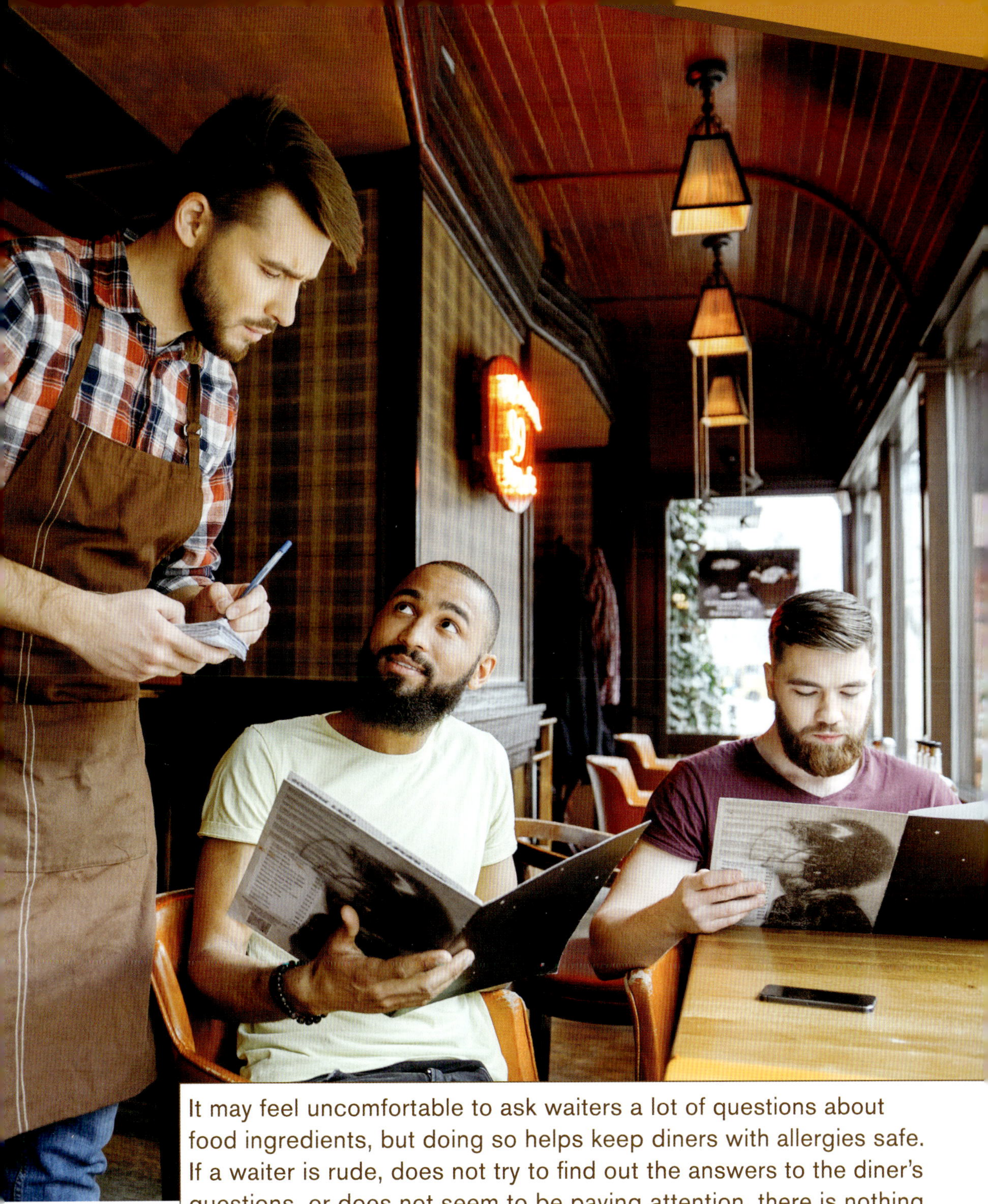

It may feel uncomfortable to ask waiters a lot of questions about food ingredients, but doing so helps keep diners with allergies safe. If a waiter is rude, does not try to find out the answers to the diner's questions, or does not seem to be paying attention, there is nothing wrong with leaving and going to a different restaurant to eat.

that should not stop you from doing so. Overall, feeling comfortable where you are is critical. If you don't get a good vibe from the people you talk to or just don't trust that the food you're getting is safe, do not eat there … Once you find a few restaurants that you feel comfortable eating at, continue eating at them. It's nice to get to know the people who work at a restaurant and develop a good relationship with them, helping you feel safe to enjoy your meal.[45]

Even after someone has found a restaurant that takes their health issues seriously, though, allergists emphasize that they have to keep their guard up. This caution is especially necessary when someone becomes comfortable with a particular restaurant chain. Writer Melissa Taylor offered this advice to other people with allergies:

If you find a local restaurant where you feel safe eating, the same chain or franchise a few miles away may have different ingredients in the exact same dish that can make you sick. Perhaps no matter where you have gone … this chain has used the same ingredients and cooking practices as the others in the chain. However, you only need to have one that doesn't handle food preparation exactly the same in order to potentially experience a reaction … Make sure you check ingredients and possible cross-contamination each and every time.[46]

Allergists often tell their patients that they can make the process of eating out much easier and safer if they prepare written materials in advance that can be shared with restaurant chefs, waiters, and waitresses. These personalized cards should include all foods and related ingredients to which the person is allergic, emergency contact information, and information on ways to avoid cross contamination.

These information cards can also include epinephrine auto-injector operating instructions in case an allergic reaction occurs and the person becomes too sick to use it themselves. "Many of my friends know where my EpiPens are and how to use them," said 16-year-old Peter, who is allergic to fish, peanuts, and tree nuts. "When I go camping, my cooking partner makes sure all the food that he provides for dinner is safe. If I were to eat a nut in the middle of a week-long canoeing trip, getting help would be a challenge … Although my friends help ensure my safety, ultimately I am responsible for my safety."[47]

Navigating Allergies with Parents

As kids grow older, they naturally seek more independence from their parents. Finding the right balance between protecting and letting go is hard enough for the parents of children who do not have any serious allergy issues. Fights may arise over the issue; for example, parents who remind their child to take their auto-injector with them may be seen as nagging and unreasonable to a teen who does not want to have to carry their auto-injector everywhere they go.

In situations where food-allergic kids clash with their parents over food rules and precautions—such as whether they should go to a party where allergenic food might be present—it is sometimes a good idea to seek the judgment of an impartial third party. According to Robert A. Wood, the family allergist is often ideally suited for this role. "Your doctor is unlikely to make the decision for you, but he may be able to defuse the emotional dynamite, highlight the facts, and explain the potential risks and rewards, so you can arrive at a more reasonable consensus," he wrote. "Some parents are far too restrictive, and teens are far too prone to taking risks. The trick is to find a happy medium."[48]

Some parents of kids with food allergies admit to feeling isolated from families that do not have to worry about food allergies. Many of them say that parents of kids without allergies simply cannot comprehend the pressure they are under every day. For example, one parent, Heather, has a young daughter, Hailey, who is severely allergic to egg and dairy products. Heather noted that she found it difficult to explain to other parents the concerns she had about Hailey's safety. Fortunately for Heather and other parents in her situation, many support groups for parents of children with severe allergies have been established. Some of these groups are community based. Others are online message boards that allow parents all around the world to talk to one another about food allergy issues. These sites can be a valuable resource for information on food allergy symptoms and treatments, menu planning tips, recipes, and strategies for navigating

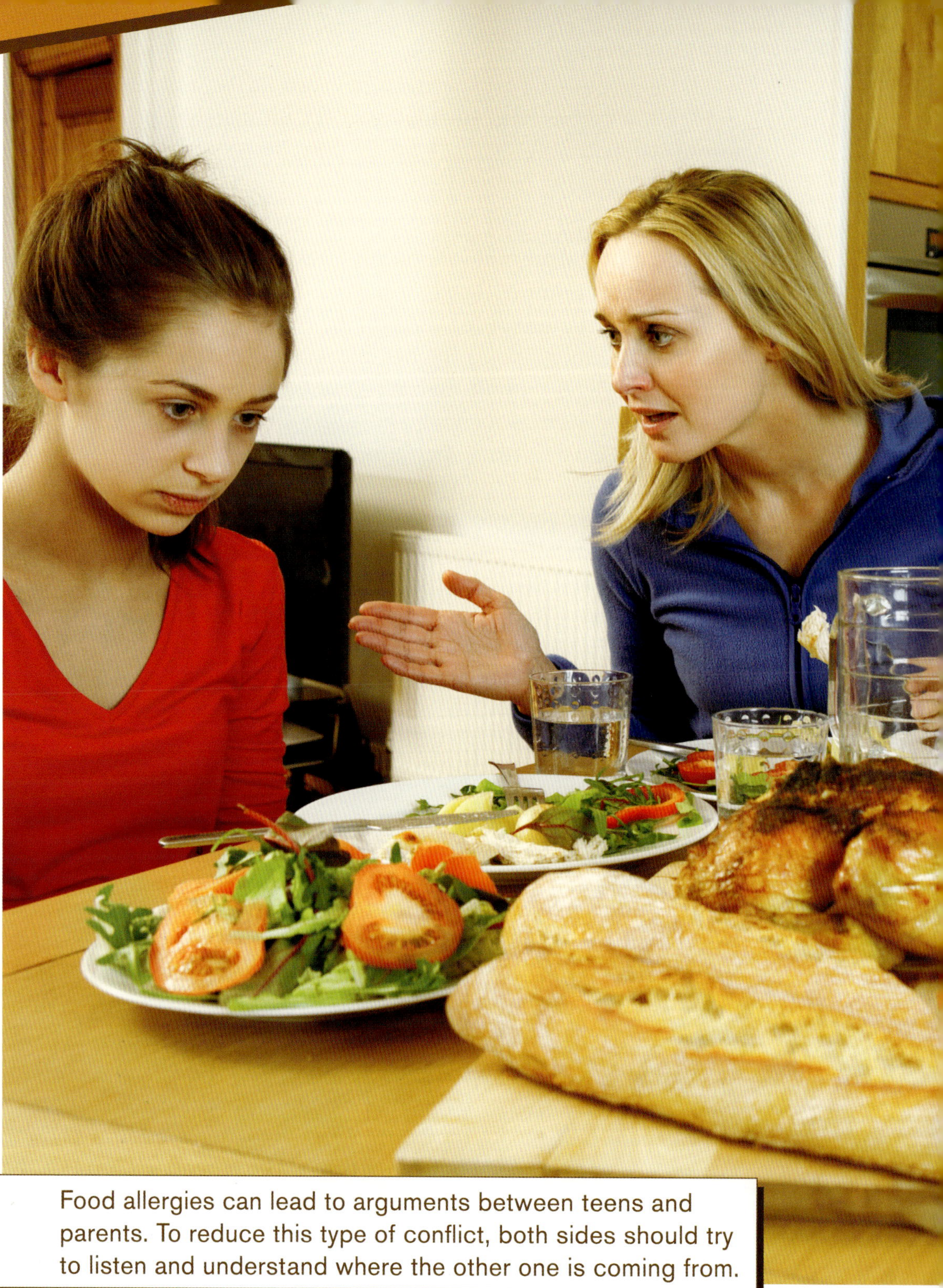

Food allergies can lead to arguments between teens and parents. To reduce this type of conflict, both sides should try to listen and understand where the other one is coming from.

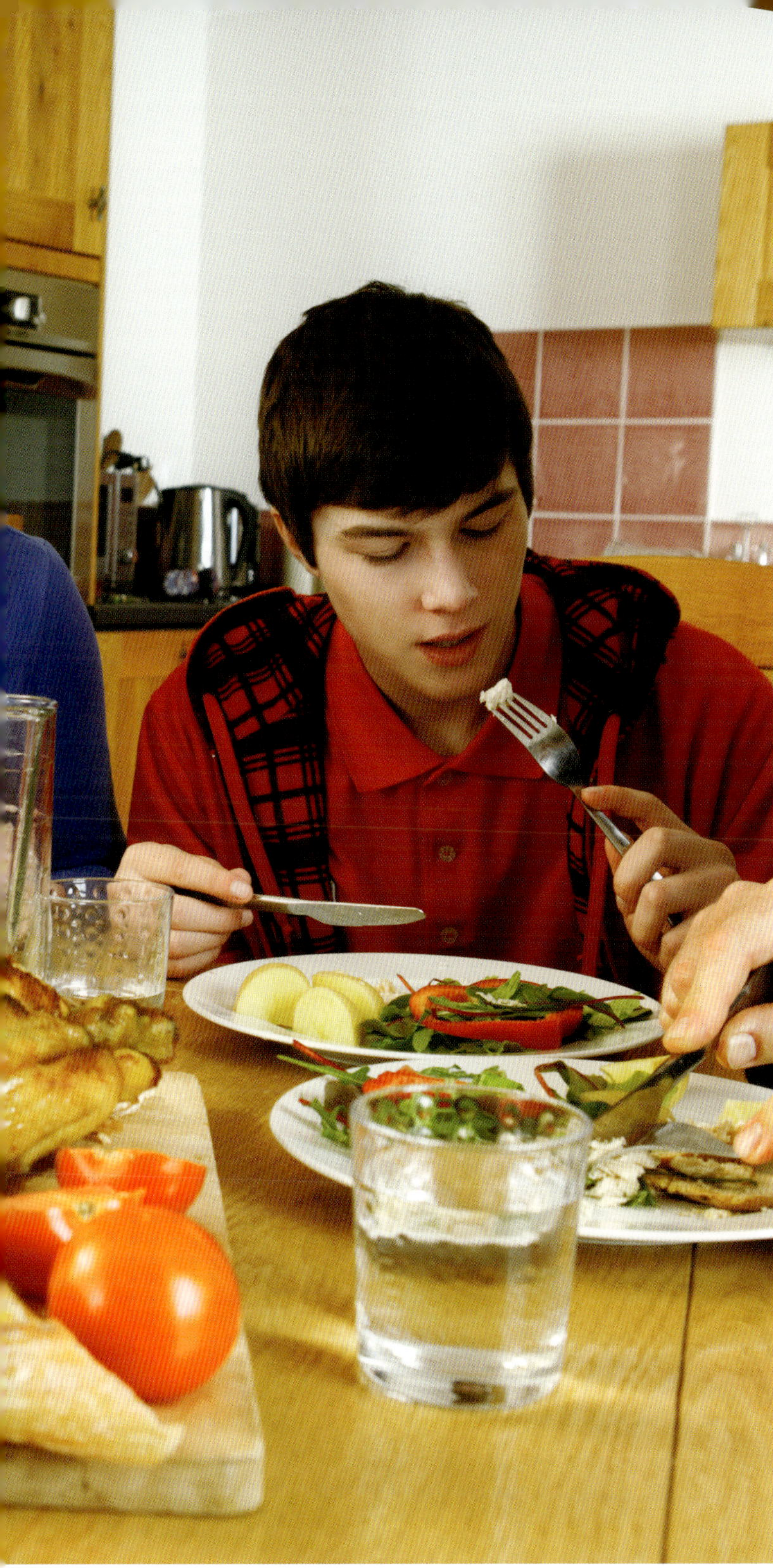

allergy challenges at home, day care, school, camp, and college.

Support networks also exist for people who are dealing with their own severe food allergies. Most of the major organizations engaged in food allergy research, education, and advocacy maintain online forums to help people with food allergies find support and encouragement. Many teen-friendly books have also been published on this subject. These works acknowledge that food allergies can be "particularly frustrating in your teenage years, when thoughts of dating and college overshadow the importance of remembering to read food labels," wrote physician Paul M. Ehrlich. "Becoming a teenager no doubt comes with increasing independence, but it is important to remember that with independence comes great responsibility, especially if you are a teen with a food allergy."[49]

Allergies Do Not Define a Person

The daily lives of individuals with severe food allergies—and their families—are full of challenges. They have to be on guard at all times against accidental exposure to potentially deadly allergens. Some activities and foods that most people take for granted are either off-limits for them or have to be undertaken with extreme caution. As a result of all these factors, people with food allergies sometimes experience embarrassment about their condition. These feelings typically reach a peak during their teen years, when many people feel intense pressure to conform to their peers and look and act like everyone else.

Despite all of these hurdles, though, millions of people of all ages who have food allergies lead rewarding and interesting lives. They play sports, travel abroad, pursue artistic or musical passions, and go to dances and parties like everyone else. They often eat well too. As Wood wrote, "clearing the cupboards of the foods that ail you doesn't condemn you to a lifetime of rice cakes and distilled water. The world offers an abundance of tasty and nutritional substitutes for the most common troublesome foods, and the food industry is pumping out more variations each year."[50]

A Closer Look

According to the CDC, although some flu vaccines are made with egg proteins, it is safe for people with an egg allergy to receive the vaccine from a health care provider who has been trained to recognize allergic reactions.

Like many people who experience a drastic change in health, those diagnosed with food allergies often find that their priorities change once the shock wears off. After learning how to eat and live in a new way, they can often laugh at many of the things that used to bother them. Problems that once seemed impossible to overcome may all of a sudden seem tiny; for example, a bad hair day pales in comparison to the memory of a severe allergic reaction. Of course, living with a severe food allergy can be tiring, and there will be times when it feels like too much to deal with. Learning to manage the stress that comes with having a food allergy is essential; taking time to do something such as meditate, watch a favorite movie, or eat a comforting food that is guaranteed not to contain an allergen can help someone feel calmer and more ready to take on the challenges life brings them.

NOTES

Introduction: Food Safety and Allergies

1. Sandra Beasley, *Don't Kill the Birthday Girl: Tales from an Allergic Life*. New York, NY: Crown, 2011, p. 4.

Chapter One: Defining Food Allergies

2. "Food Allergies," KidsHealth, last updated August 2018. kidshealth.org/en/kids/food-allergies.html#.
3. Robert A. Wood and Joe Kraynak, *Food Allergies for Dummies*. Indianapolis, IN: Wiley, 2007, p. 12.
4. Laura Beil, "Little by Little: As Food Allergies Proliferate, New Strategies May Help Patients Ingest Their Way to Tolerance," *Science News*, September 12, 2009, p. 20.
5. Susan Dominus, "The Allergy Prison," *New York Times*, June 10, 2001. www.nytimes.com/2001/06/10/magazine/the-allergy-prison.html.
6. Quoted in Dominus, "The Allergy Prison."
7. Dan Mangan, "Mylan Hit with Racketeering Suit over Big Price Hikes of EpiPen," CNBC, April 3, 2017. www.cnbc.com/2017/04/03/mylan-hit-with-racketeering-suit-over-big-price-hikes-of-epipen.html.
8. Elizabeth Landau, "Allergy Injectors are Liberating and Daunting," CNN, September 4, 2009. www.cnn.com/2009/HEALTH/09/04/food.allergies.bees.epipen/index.html.
9. Wood and Kraynak, *Food Allergies for Dummies*, p. 53.

Chapter Two: Food Allergies on the Rise

10. Claudia Kalb, "Fear and Allergies in the Lunchroom," *Newsweek*, October 27, 2007. www.newsweek.com/fear-and-allergies-lunchroom-103015.

11. Quoted in Dominus, "The Allergy Prison."

12. Quoted in Sarah Boseley, "Bogus Allergy Tests Causing Real Harm, Say Experts," *Guardian*, June 4, 2015. www.theguardian.com/society/2015/jun/04/bogus-allergy-tests-causing-real-harm-say-experts.

13. Beil, "Little by Little," p. 20.

14. Elisa Meyer, *Feeding Your Allergic Child: Happy Food for Healthy Kids*. New York, NY: St. Martin's Press, 1997, pp. 9–10.

15. Joanna Blythman, "Are We Really Wrong to Blame Processed Food for the Rise in Allergies?," *Guardian*, June 5, 2015. www.theguardian.com/commentisfree/2015/jun/05/blame-processed-food-rise-in-allergies.

16. Jamie Ducharme, "Millions of People Wrongly Believe They Have Food Allergies," *TIME*, January 8, 2019. time.com/5497070/food-allergy-intolerance/.

17. Ducharme, "Millions of People Wrongly Believe."

18. "Study: Food Allergies on Rise in U.S. Kids," CBS News, October 22, 2008. www.cbsnews.com/news/study-food-allergies-on-rise-in-us-kids/.

19. Tim Yeomans, "Does Being Too Clean Cause Allergies?," Allergy Standards, July 13, 2018. www.allergystandards.com/news_events/hygiene-hypothesis/.

20. Quoted in "C-Section Babies' Immune System May Be Improved by Vaginal Microbial Transfer," University of Utah Health, February 25, 2016. healthcare.utah.edu/the-scope/shows.php?shows=0_8jtrca8z.

21. Yeomans, "Does Being Too Clean Cause Allergies?"

22. Quoted in Sarah Abo, "Asian Environment May Protect Children Against Nut Allergies: Study," SBS News, February 17, 2016. www.sbs.com.au/news/asian-environment-may-protect-children-against-nut-allergies-study.

Chapter Three: Identifying a Food Allergy

23. "Food Allergies," KidsHealth.

24. Quoted in William E. Walsh, *Food Allergies: The Complete Guide to Understanding and Relieving Your Food Allergies*. New York, NY: John Wiley, 2000.

25. "Food Allergy Overview," AAAAI, accessed on April 12, 2019. www.aaaai.org/conditions-and-treatments/allergies/food-allergies.

26. "Skin Prick Tests," FARE, accessed on April 12, 2019. www.foodallergy.org/life-with-food-allergies/food-allergy-101/diagnosis-testing/skin-prick-tests.

27. "Blood Tests," FARE, accessed on April 12, 2019. www.foodallergy.org/life-with-food-allergies/food-allergy-101/diagnosis-testing/blood-tests.

28. Quoted in Melinda Beck, "New Rules for Food Allergies," *Wall Street Journal*, December 7, 2010. www.wsj.com/articles/SB10001424052748704156304576003382894873452.

Chapter Four: Laws, Science, and Food Production

29. Tess O'Brien-Heinzen, "A Complex Recipe: Food Allergies and the Law," *Wisconsin Lawyer*, May 2010. www.wisbar.org/NewsPublications/WisconsinLawyer/Pages/Article.aspx?ArticleID=1876.

30. O'Brien-Heinzen, "A Complex Recipe."

31. Quoted in "Food Allergy Management Act Becomes Law," Barney Butter, January 5, 2011. barneybutter.com/food-allergy-management-act-becomes-law/.

32. "What Happens to Food Allergies After Treatment with Oral Immunotherapy?," AAAAI, March 2016. www.aaaai.org/about-aaaai/newsroom/news-releases/food-allergy-oral-immunotherapy.

33. Quoted in Beil, "Little by Little," p. 20.

34. Wood and Kraynak, *Food Allergies for Dummies*, p. 162.

35. Kalb, "Fear and Allergies in the Lunchroom."

36. Kevin T. Higgins, "Allergens and Labeling: Got It Under Control?," *Food Engineering*, March 6, 2006.

37. Quoted in Higgins, "Allergens and Labeling: Got It Under Control?"

Chapter Five: Living Life to Its Fullest

38. Quoted in Lianne Mandelbaum, "28 Things People with Food Allergies Wish You Knew," The Mighty, September 6, 2018. themighty.com/2018/09/food-allergies-what-its-like/.
39. Quoted in Mary Brophy Marcus, "Food Allergy Sufferers Find Socializing Tricky," *USA Today*, January 7, 2010. www.usatoday.com/news/health/2010-01-07-allergies07_CV_N.htm.
40. Annie Jorgensen, "A Message from Miss Wisconsin's Outstanding Teen 2011," FAAN Teen, accessed on May 9, 2019. www.faanteen.org/personalstories/miss_outstanding_teen_message.php.
41. "Telling My Teammates About My Food Allergies," FAAN Teen, accessed on May 9, 2019. www.faanteen.org/school/teammates.php.
42. Nicole Smith, "Food Allergy Anxiety," AllergicChild, November 27, 2017. home.allergicchild.com/category/emotional-aspects-of-food-allergies/.
43. "Food Allergies," KidsHealth.
44. Pete Wells, "Beating Eggs," *New York Times*, March 3, 2009. www.nytimes.com/2009/03/08/magazine/08food-t-000.html.
45. "A Successful Night Out," FAAN Teen, accessed on May 9, 2019. www.faanteen.org/personalstories/night_out.php.
46. Melissa Taylor, *Food Allergy Survivors Together Handbook*. San Jose, CA: Writers Club, 2002, p. 42.
47. "A Whole Lotta Love," FAAN Teen, accessed on May 9, 2019. www.faanteen.org/personalstories/lotta_love.php.
48. Wood and Kraynak, *Food Allergies for Dummies*, p. 244.
49. Paul M. Ehrlich and Elizabeth Shimer Bowers, *Living with Allergies*. New York, NY: Facts On File, 2009, p. 102.
50. Wood and Kraynak, *Food Allergies for Dummies*, p. 287.

ORGANIZATIONS TO CONTACT

American Academy of Allergy, Asthma & Immunology (AAAAI)
555 East Wells Street, Suite 1100
Milwaukee, WI 53202
www.aaaai.org
twitter.com/AAAAI_org

This organization works to educate the public about all kinds of allergies, including food allergies.

Asthma and Allergy Foundation of America (AAFA)
201 Corporate Drive, Suite 1000
Landover, MD 20785
www.aafa.org
twitter.com/AAFANational
www.youtube.com/user/ForLifeWithoutLimits

AAFA provides educational information and community-based services to people in the United States through regional chapters and support groups. The group also funds research into allergy treatment and cures.

Food Allergy Research & Education (FARE)
7901 Jones Branch Drive, Suite 240
McLean, VA 22102
www.foodallergy.org
www.instagram.com/foodallergy
twitter.com/FoodAllergy
www.youtube.com/user/FAANPAL

FARE is a multifaceted advocacy organization that plays a leading role in educating Americans about food allergies and anaphylaxis.

Kids with Food Allergies Foundation
4259 West Swamp Road, Suite 408
Doylestown, PA 18902
www.kidswithfoodallergies.org
twitter.com/kfatweets
www.youtube.com/user/KFAAdmin

This division of AAFA provides educational information on all aspects of coping with food allergies. Its webiste includes a directory of food recipes searchable by allergens that commonly need to be avoided.

FOR MORE INFORMATION

Books

Coss, Linda Marienhoff. *What's to Eat?: The Milk-Free, Egg-Free, Nut-Free Food Allergy Cookbook*. Lake Forest, CA: Plumtree Press, 2017.
This popular recipe book contains instructions for making more than 145 meals and desserts that are free of dairy, egg, and nut allergens.

Deldicque, Olivier. *When Every Bite Matters: One Teen's Journey with Food Allergies*. Fayetteville, NY: Pop Fly Publishing, 2018.
This book offers lifesaving advice from a teen's perspective.

Gulati, Annette. *Life with Food Allergies*. Mankato, MN: Child's World, 2019.
This book takes a look at the everyday lives of people with food allergies.

Reino, Jessica. *Food Allergies: The Ultimate Teen Guide*. Lanham, MD: Rowman & Littlefield, 2017.
Teens with allergies can use this guide to learn how to take charge of their health by advocating for themselves and cooking well despite their dietary restrictions.

Sicherer, Scott H. *Food Allergies: A Complete Guide for Eating When Your Life Depends on It*. Baltimore, MD: John Hopkins University Press, 2017.
This is a comprehensive guide to learning how to manage food allergies.

Websites

Allergy Haven

www.allergyhaven.com

Founded by the mother of a child with food allergies, this website's mission is to educate and empower people who live with food allergies.

FDA: What You Need to Know about Food Allergies

www.fda.gov/Food/IngredientsPackagingLabeling/FoodAllergens/ucm079311.htm

This section of the website of the Food and Drug Administration (FDA) provides consumers with basic background information on food allergies and explains the FDA's role in ensuring the safety of people with allergies.

KidsHealth: Food Allergies

kidshealth.org/kid/ill_injure/sick/food_allergies.html#

This section of the KidsHealth website provides a kid-friendly explanation of how food allergies work. It also includes tips on how people with food allergies can adjust their diets.

Medline Plus: Food Allergy

medlineplus.gov/foodallergy.html

This website, which is maintained by the National Institutes of Health, offers a wide range of information on food allergy issues.

TeensHealth: Allergies

kidshealth.org/en/teens/allergies.html

People are allergic to many things besides food. This website gives a general overview of allergies and helpful information, such as how to prepare for an allergy emergency.

INDEX

PICTURE CREDITS

Cover Image Point Fr/Shutterstock.com; p. 7 Africa Studio/Shutterstock.com; p. 10 THPStock/Shutterstock.com; p. 15 chomplearn/Shutterstock.com; pp. 18–19 Erik McGregor/Pacific Press/LightRocket via Getty Images; pp. 20–21 bitt24/Shutterstock.com; p. 23 BELIMBINGperak/Shutterstock.com; pp. 24–25 cobraphotography/Shutterstock.com; p. 30 New Africa/Shutterstock.com; p. 32 Everett Historical/Shutterstock.com; pp. 35, 88–89 Monkey Business Images/Shutterstock.com; pp. 36–37 ESB Professional/Shutterstock.com; p. 43 XiXinXing/Shutterstock.com; pp. 46–47 BSIP/UIG via Getty Images; pp. 50–51 Lipik Stock Media/Shutterstock.com; p. 53 tarapong srichaiyos/Shutterstock.com; p. 56 OPOLJA/Shutterstock.com; p. 57 Odua Images/Shutterstock.com; pp. 60–61 Ruslan Galiullin/Shutterstock.com; pp. 64–65 Robert Willet/The News & Observer/TNS via Getty Images; pp. 66–67 wavebreakmedia/Shutterstock.com; pp. 68–69 Moshbidon/Shutterstock.com; pp. 70–71 David Tonelson/Shutterstock.com; p. 75 Iakov Filimonov/Shutterstock.com; p. 79 EvgeniiAnd/Shutterstock.com; pp. 80–81 Melinda Nagy/Shutterstock.com; pp. 82–83 Norb_KM/Shutterstock.com; pp. 84–85 Dean Drobot/Shutterstock.com.

ABOUT THE AUTHOR

Jason Brainard received a B.A. in anthropology and an M.A. in English from SUNY at Fredonia. He currently lives in the beautiful Hudson Valley with his wonderful wife and two daughters. Jason developed an allergy to tree nuts when he was 39. It was a bummer. However, he has since learned to appreciate the nuances of many exotic cheeses.